I0479308

Amazing Twists of the Mind

BY

NASH N. BOUTROS, MD

Copyright © 2023 by Nash N. Boutros, MD
All rights reserved.

Dedication

I dedicate this book to all my patients and their families. They taught me a lot not only about my profession but also about life. I also dedicate this book to all those professionals who dedicate their lives to helping individuals suffering from severe psychiatric disorders. They are heroes working with very little and trying to accomplish so much.

Table of Contents

Glossary of Terms and Abbreviations

Conversion Disorders: When a patient presents with a neurological complaint (like weakness on one side, blindness, or seizures) but the physician finds no evidence from the clinical examination or any tests for actual neurological damage. The term is used mainly by psychiatrists and other mental health workers. The term used by neurologists is "Functional Neurological Disorders".

DSM: Diagnostic and Statistical Manual of Mental Disorders. The DSM is a book that is published by the American Psychiatric Association and lists the diagnostic criteria of all currently known psychiatric disorders. It is constantly evolving and is now in its fifth edition (DSM-5).

EEG: Electroencephalography. The measurement and study of the brain's electrical activity. A commonly used term is Brainwave testing. This is the only widely available method to test for epileptic activity. EEG can also detect other forms of brain dysfunction.

MEG: Magnetoencephalography. The measurement and study of the brain's magnetic activity. This is a seriously more expensive test, and its availability is limited to research institutions. The brain's magnetic activity is much weaker than the electrical activity and requires very special equipment to be able to detect it which necessitates that it be shielded from the huge earth's magnetic field. Nonetheless, it can see deeper into the brain and can detect activity coming from smaller structures.

Neuropsychology testing: This can be a paper and pencil test, or computer-administered. It is designed to test for cognitive dysfunctions. It is widely used in Neurology practices but its use in Psychiatry remains limited.

Neuropsychiatry: A subspecialty of psychiatry where patients with neurological disorders and psychiatric complications (e.g., epilepsy and depression) can find expert help.

Psychotherapy: Psychotherapy is a form of treatment for psychiatric disorders that relies mainly on talk therapy and psychological exercises. It has many forms like Cognitive Behavioral Therapy (CBT) and Psychoanalysis. Supportive psychotherapy entails providing support and education to patients and their families. This form of therapy is provided essentially by all medical practitioners. The other forms of psychotherapy like CBT require extensive training.

TMS: Transcranial Magnetic Stimulation. TMS is an emerging technology that allows the modulation of the activity of a specific area of the brain. It is non-invasive. A magnetic stimulation coil is placed on the scalp to target an area of the brain and is then discharged. It is by and far not painful.

INTRODUCTION

As a life-long learner, I took every opportunity to learn from any person or situation that I encountered. Some of my most significant learning experiences came from my encounters with those individuals who sought my professional help as a psychiatrist. In this book, I recount twenty-eight of the most enlightening experiences I had during my 50-year career. **All personal and identifying information was altered to protect the identity of the actual patients.** The most interesting aspect of the case was taken, and an entirely fictional character and circumstances were built on it. Any similarity with any person's condition is simply the reflection that such afflictions are not uncommon. The figures are the workings of the imagination of the artist. I hope you will find the stories interesting, entertaining, and educational.

Early on in my life, I was faced with the tragic loss of my baby sister. She had a disorder that had no-effective treatment at the time. At age eleven, I was asking everyone, including my learned parents and college-age brothers, why should this happen. I was given the answer that was "God's will" and that I should not be asking such questions. Only a few years later, treatment for this disorder was discovered and became available. There was no doubt in my young mind that my sister died because SCIENCE has not provided the answer when she needed it. Were the answers available, she would not have died. All other explanations paled in comparison to this explanation. From this point forward, I firmly subscribed to the power of science in solving all our problems. All my subsequent readings and experiences simply confirmed this belief.

As part of the medical school curriculum, I had to study Human Physiology. The textbook of human physiology that was assigned was comprised of six volumes. One entire volume was dedicated to the nervous system. I was fascinated by it. It was so complex that one could not help but be amazed by it. As I have already decided to pursue a research career, this system (i.e., The Central Nervous System or CNS) seemed to be much more wide-open for investigations. Hence my decision to dedicate my career to studying the workings of the brain.

Then I arrived at my Psychiatry rotation during my internship. I had a wonderful mentor, Professor Mohamed Shaalan who was US-trained and at the cutting edge of the field. He also strongly subscribed to the power of science. During this rotation, I faced the case that shaped my career, Case # one in the book. It immediately made me recognize the degree of ignorance the field was swimming in. I decided that any contribution I make to shed any degree of light on any of the psychiatric disorders would be a significant contribution. I also had my Neurology rotation. Fascinating as neurological disorders are, there was more known about them with already significant ongoing research. Nonetheless, my fascination with all brain disorders continued and I had to make up my mind about which way to go.

The final and deciding step came during my year of advanced training in Behavioral Neurology and Epilepsy in Dallas, Texas. It so happened that during this fellowship year, the two large annual meetings of the two disciplines; the American Psychiatric Association (APA) and the American Academy of Neurology (AAN) were being held in Dallas. I attended both meetings. The APA conference went on for five days, from seven AM to 8-9 PM daily with almost 12-14 simultaneous presentations at any one time. The breadth of topics to be covered was amazingly vast. In contrast, the AAN was a significantly smaller meeting. I guess I had already made up my mind at this point.

Starting from the events around the tragic loss of my sister and many subsequent events and the many books I had access to, I found myself deviating from the Christian Orthodoxy belief system I was born into and arrived at Secular Humanism. Details of this journey are recounted in my autobiography (A Journey from Orthodoxy to Humanism; We are not alone). The ways Humanist ideals affected my thinking about Psychiatry are detailed in "Humanist Psychiatry, 2nd Edition).

Humanism is optimistic regarding human nature and confident in human reason and Science as the best means of reaching the goal of human fulfillment in this world. Humanists affirm that humans are a product of the same evolutionary process that produced all other organisms and that all ideas, knowledge, values, and social systems are based upon human experience. Humanists conclude that creative ability and personal responsibility are strongest when the mind is free from supernatural beliefs and operates in an atmosphere of freedom and democracy.

To summarize, Humanist Psychiatry is based on the following four general principles:

1) That every effort should be made to alleviate the suffering of humans afflicted with psychiatric disorders. This includes providing the best treatment available at the time and maximizing the scientific search for further understanding and treatment of psychiatric disorders.

2) That our knowledge of the causes and treatments of psychiatric disorders remains minimal as evidenced by the lack of any proven etiology of any of the diseases included in the Diagnostic and Statistical Manual (DSM) published by the American Psychiatric Association and now in its fifth edition (DSM-5). Moreover, while many of the symptoms of psychiatric disorders can be temporarily brought under control, no known cure exists for any of these disorders.

3) The third principle is that advancing knowledge regarding the brain, its physiology, anatomy, chemistry, genetics, and the impact of social interactions (including trauma and abuse) on all these areas is essential for the eventual understanding and effective treatment of such disorders.

4) The final principle is that all disorders are considered biological (i.e., brain disorders) in origin until proven otherwise. This is in total opposition to current attitudes where if there is no readily apparent biological correlate the disorder is considered "psychological" or a disorder of the mind and not the brain.

The cases I chose to include in this book have specific messages to learners and the public. I included the diagnostic criteria for some of the cases for educational purposes, but my takes and the special messages/significance are included under "My Thoughts" at the end of the cases.

References:

Nash N Boutros. A Journey from Orthodoxy to Humanism; We are not alone. Amazon.com, 2022.

Boutros NN. Humanist Psychiatry, 2nd edition. Nova Science Publishers. 2022. New York. ISBN: 978-1-68507-501-9

Kurtz, Pal.2000. The Humanist Manifesto 2000. Prometheus Books; Amherst, New York. (Kurtz, 2000).

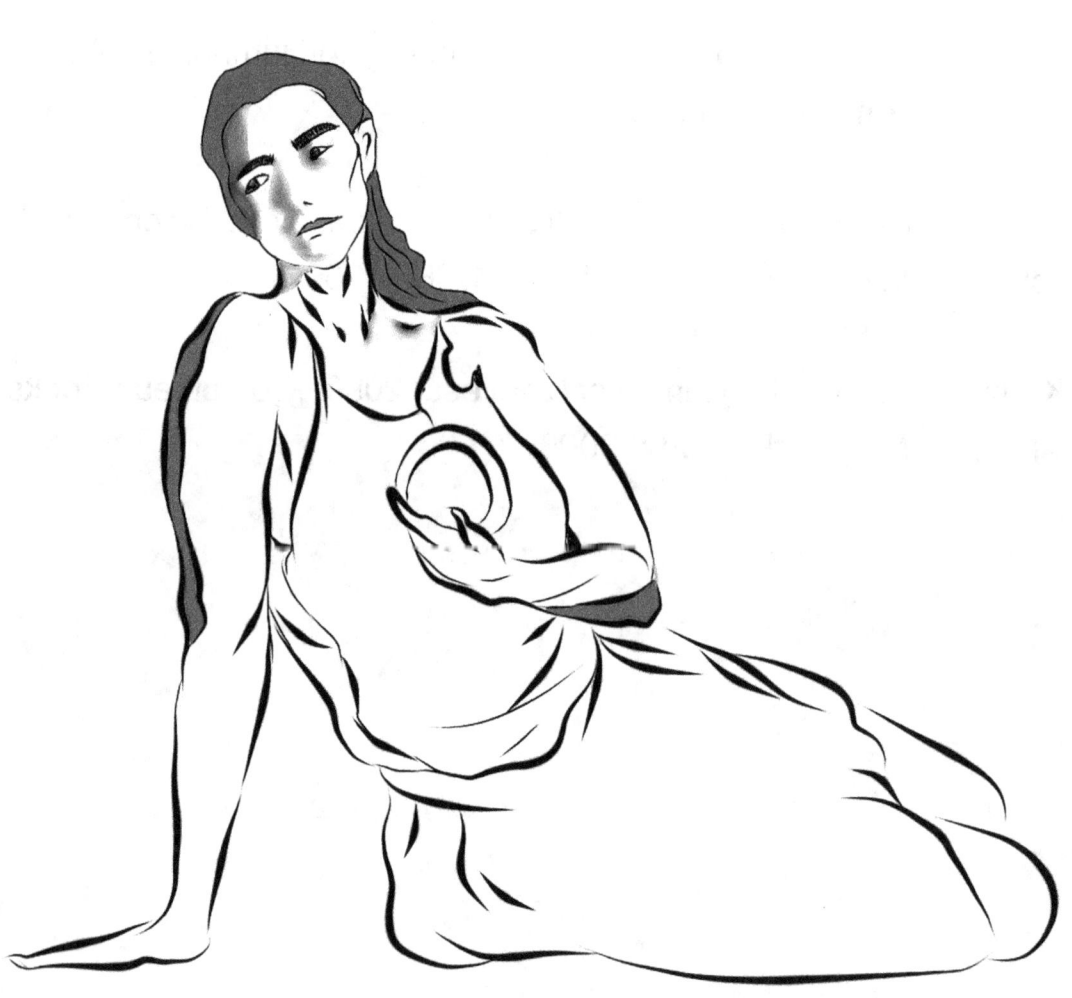

Case One
The Case That Got It All Started

The setting was the Outpatient Clinic of the Psychiatry Department at Cairo University Hospital in 1974. It was during my clinical rotation into the psychiatry portion of my one-year internship. While drawn to Psychiatry, I had not made a final commitment to it due to my increasing fascination with the field of Neurology. My indecision about a career choice came to an end one morning when I was asked to see a 17-year-old girl. I was not told what the reason was for her visit to the clinic.

When the clinic assistant gave me the patient's name, I expected that one of her parents would escort her, given her young age. I had no idea what was waiting for me or what I was about to experience: my first face-to-face encounter with the enormity of the diagnostic and healing tasks at hand. The clinic assistant opened the door and ushered in the girl and her parents. The mother, a well-dressed, middle-class woman walked in first, followed by her daughter, with the father trailing behind. Also well-dressed, middle class, and with glasses.

My first impression was that of a solid middle-class family. I welcomed the patient and her parents and asked them to be seated. Looking at the mother, I inquired what had brought them to the clinic that morning. The mother promptly asked the father to leave the room, and he calmly complied. Once he had left, the mother asked her daughter – I will call her Bella- to disrobe. What I saw then, and what I soon learned about the limitations of diagnosis in the field of psychiatry, would soon clear up my indecision about the career path I wanted.

1

Disrobed, Bella had razor cuts covering her arms and upper thighs. Cigarette burns were spotted in her abdominal area. The briefest inspection sufficed for me to see the severity of Bella's issues. I asked her to put her clothes back on. I looked at the mother and asked her to tell me what had happened.

The mother, now sobbing, said simply that her daughter – her only child – had started exhibiting this self-mutilating behavior a year ago for no obvious reason besides the stress of a difficult school year. But a stressful school year was unlikely to be the cause of such self-destructive behavior. I started probing for stressful experiences in Bella's earlier life. The mother stated clearly, and convincingly, that she was unaware of further stresses. I learned that Bella's father was a prominent lawyer. The family had no financial problems. The mother insisted that he was an exemplary father who showered attention and care on both of them. Bella nodded in full agreement.

Psychiatrists consider the symptom of self-mutilation, when not linked to suicidal intent, to be the hallmark of the syndrome of borderline personality disorder (BPD). Later, that afternoon and well into the evening, I was in the medical school library. I found many books about BPD and began reading them. All of them. Six days later, I learned much of what psychiatry had to say about BPD and how it tried to help patients suffering from it. This reading was a rude awakening.

Psychiatry, it turned out, couldn't do much. It diagnosed BPD only as resulting from some form of child abuse, with the father being the likely offender. The best treatment it could offer was years of costly and inconclusive psychotherapy, for which I was unqualified at the time. In Bella's case, I had seen little evidence of abuse in this apparently caring family or among Bella's friends. In all of my readings about BPD, there was no mention of the possible involvement of the brain in this disorder.

The time for a second appointment came, and the family showed up as expected. I started by asking both the father and the patient to leave the room. I then turned my attention to the mother and began probing for any possible grounds for the possibility of any form of abuse including sexual abuse by the father or any other male member of the family or any other acquaintances considered close friends. The mother was clear and forceful in denying this possibility. I had not expected this response. I told the mother that sexual abuse was the prevailing and in fact *only* theory in cases like Bella's, but she doubled down on the impossibility of abuse in any way, form, or shape.

But the mother did tell me something new. Bella had a pattern of loving her close friends intensely but then suddenly turning on them for no clear reason. It was at these times of emotional tension, she said, that Bella's cutting behaviors would increase. Bella herself later told me that her self-hurting behaviors gave her relief from anxiety. But not much, for constantly she worried that in the end, her friends would all leave her. Indeed, she said she didn't have that many friends left. Yet surprisingly, Bella denied almost all symptoms indicative of a major depressive disorder. I had no compelling reason to doubt her report.

In the coming week, preparing for the third and final visit with the family, I continued probing the library for all available knowledge about BPD and the sexual abuse theory. I found many opinions and judgments, but nothing convincing, nothing based on science. In the end, I had to conclude that BPD had yet to be scientifically studied, and worse yet, that experimental research into it was almost entirely lacking.

The field of psychiatry, I reluctantly decided, treats what it doesn't understand with unproven methods that offer little promise of a cure. This sad conclusion led to my career decision to pursue research into the biological basis of psychiatric disorders following a well-accepted scientific research methodology. And it led to another decision, namely, to find training at an advanced research institution committed to the search for scientifically based cures to severe disorders like the one from which Bella suffered, along with her family.

In my third and find meeting with the family, I shared everything I had learned in my research about BPD and, having no other option, referred them to a psychotherapist known for treating this disorder. With regret, I told them that this was the best I could do. I wished them good luck. It was not a happy experience. But for me, at least, it was a learning one. To this day I wonder how life worked out for Bella and her family.

DSM-5

DSM-5 States that borderline personality disorder is characterized by some or all of these symptoms:

- Fear of abandonment and its avoidance
- Interpersonal relationships instability

- Identity disturbance
- Impulsivity
- Suicidal and self-harm behavior
- Affective instability
- Chronic feelings of emptiness
- Inappropriate intense anger
- Stress-related paranoid ideations

My Thoughts:

In my early years of medical school and until I met with Bella and her family, I had been taught to believe that psychiatric disorders (or mental conditions) are purely *mental*. That meant they result from a patient's psychological responses to events, like sexual abuse, occurring in the external world. I took this to mean that psychiatry saw nothing at all dysfunctional in the brain or other bodily systems. Seeing the severity of the symptoms presented by Bella and finding no indication anywhere of abuse of any kind, there was no doubt in my mind that something was very wrong with the brain function of this poor girl. Even today, neuroscience has yet to find any major clues into the underlying brain pathology of this devastating condition. This is sad to report. But I remain convinced that neuroscience one day will understand BPD and hopefully find a cure or at least a remediation for it.

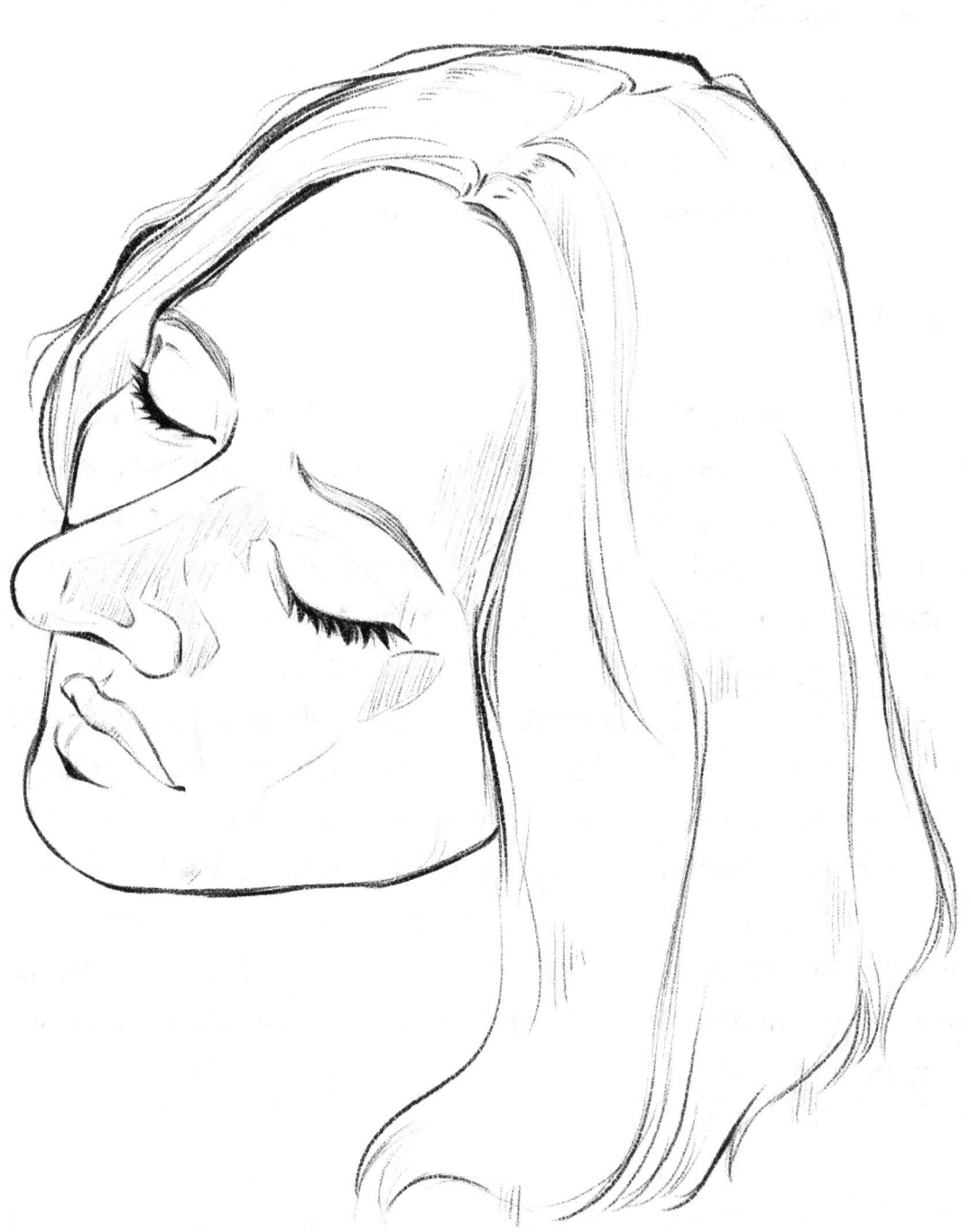

Case Two

The Lady with the Big Nose Teaches Me a Lesson. Early in My Career.

I was a third-year psychiatry resident. Each resident had to carry several patients on each of the three tracks of psychotherapy training: psychoanalysis, cognitive-behavioral therapy (CBT), and supportive therapy. Each track was supervised by a professor skilled in the appropriate psychotherapy modality. On my CBT track, I saw Ms. Nuveen. She was 25 years of age, single, and fully employed, with a mid-level [two years of college] education. From the very beginning, her problem was apparent. She had a rather unsightly big nose. She said she hated herself because of her nose and believed that it was causing her to have no dates or boyfriends. She felt isolated and alone. She was desperate.

All sessions with Ms. Nuveen were recorded for review during the supervision session. The professor/supervisor had no problem identifying her problem as a self-image issue and advised me to help Ms. Nuveen change her self-image to be more accepting of herself as she was. Her long nose would stay as it was. My job was to identify where her thought processes had gone wrong and help her redirect her thoughts so as not to blame her nose for her problems and instead to accept herself as more attractive than what she had led herself to believe.

I went to work. We had weekly sessions. She always showed up on time, well-dressed, and with make-up on. Every session revealed more about her thinking processes, which I took back to my professor-supervisor. After ten sessions, it seemed that she was beginning to come around. I began to feel good about her case. I was getting valuable training. My confidence was building up.

But the eleventh session didn't go so well. She walked in in-tears. She had just had another dating experience that ended like all the others. With her alone. She said she did not feel any better and felt she was wasting her time and mine as well. I reassured her that she was in fact doing better and urged her to hold on and persevere with her therapy. As always, I took the recording to my professor-supervisor. I was hoping that I had made a mistake of some kind that had led to this setback, one that he could help me correct to the benefit of the patient. Without faulting my work, he simply indicated that patient setbacks do occur and that I should not be discouraged but continue the prescribed therapeutic approach with Ms. Nuveen.

On week twelve - three months of therapy – Ms. Nuveen showed up in better spirits. I felt relieved. I shared with her my supervisor's ideas and suggestions. But she was surprisingly quiet, just nodding to whatever I said. I clearly indicated my full support and availability for her to call or come in more frequently if she felt the need. She smiled in appreciation.

In week thirteen, however, Ms. Nuveen was a no-show with no call to explain her absence. I asked the department secretary to call her to make sure she was OK. No response. I was now worried even though she had never indicated that she might be suicidal. All I could do at this point was to send her a certified letter with a return receipt request reminding her of the next appointment. We got the acknowledgment of receipt back, but with no further response.

Four months passed. One day, the department secretary informed me that Ms. Nuveen had made an appointment to see me. I was very glad at the news. I reviewed the tapes and my supervisor's suggestions, getting ready to resume CBT.

She showed up, as always, on time with makeup on and as always well-dressed. But this time with an obvious difference. Her nose looked fine! She had had cosmetic surgery. She looked better, happier. And she began the session with a surprise. She asked me how *I* was doing. The patient caring for the doctor! She was smiling big. And feeling good about herself.

Dr. Boutros, she said in a very affirmative and confident voice "I am here to let you know that all I needed was a nose job".

She continued, "I know you were sincere in your attempt to help me. It seemed that you believed what you were telling me. But I just wanted to contribute to your education because I think you will be a good doctor". She concluded, "What they teach here is bullshit. All I needed was this nose job".

The time soon came to share this development with my professor-supervisor. He smiled knowingly and indicated that surgery was a temporary, superficial solution that overlooked the "real," deeper issues. He predicted that Ms. Nuveen will be back with a different body part preoccupation in a few weeks.

Based on this prediction, I asked Ms. Nuveen if she would be willing to continue to see me for follow-ups once monthly. She agreed. After a year of monthly follow-up sessions, she was doing well. No bodily or mental complaints. Her social life was beginning to flourish!

Wow. That, in a word, was my reaction. Did Ms. Nuveen teach me a lesson? You bet she did, and a big one too (pun intended). I am grateful to her.

DSM-5. The standard psychiatric diagnosis of Ms. Nuveen's situation was Body Dysmorphic Disorder (BDD). It has four criteria

- Preoccupation with one or more perceived defects or flaws in physical appearance that are not observable or appear slight to others.
- At some point during the disorder, the individual has performed repetitive behaviors (e.g., mirror checking, excessive grooming, skin picking, reassurance seeking) or mental acts (e.g., comparing his or her appearance with that of others) in response to the appearance concerns.
- The preoccupation causes clinically significant distress or impairment in social, occupational, or other areas of functioning.
- The appearance preoccupation is not better explained by concerns with body fat or weight in an individual whose symptoms meet diagnostic criteria for an eating disorder.

My Thoughts:

Of course, I noted the big nose from the very first session. It was clearly very observable and more than that off-putting to many, especially to possible suitors. Sensing this I empathized with the patient. However, the idea of suggesting that she go for cosmetic surgery never crossed my mind. I did eventually run it by my professor-supervisor, but he said he thought it was a naïve idea.

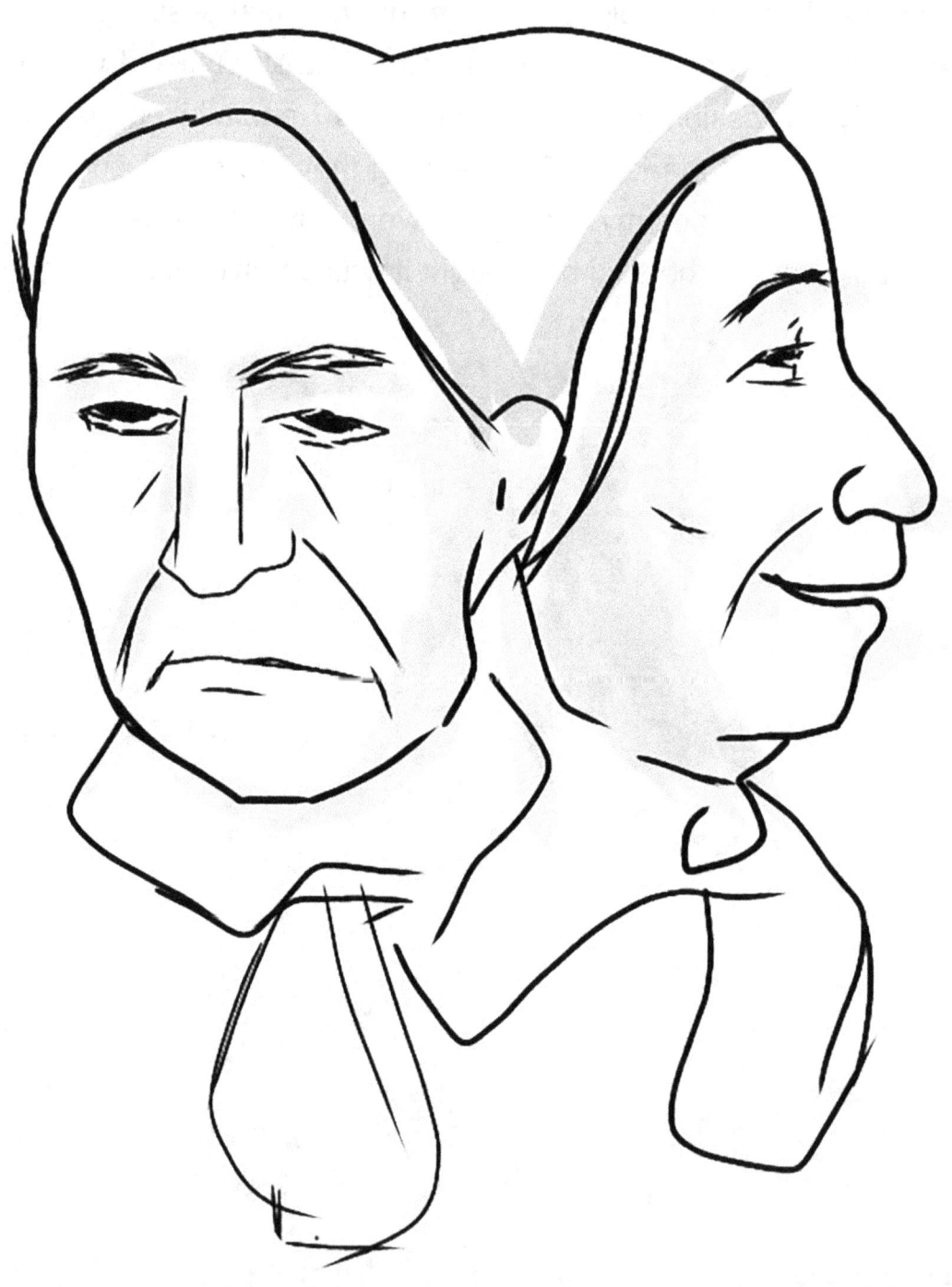

Case Three

Laughing and Crying but Neither Happy nor Sad!

I was a junior faculty member at a midsize medical school. In this position, I had a joint appointment between the departments of Psychiatry and Neurology. My caseload included a good number of elderly patients who usually had cognitive problems, but Ms. Patricia was my first case with this problem. I was asked to see this patient for evaluation of either major depression or bipolar disorder. The consultation stated that Ms. Patricia, a 74-year-old woman, had at times been observed crying and at other times laughing for no clear reason. She had been admitted to the hospital for evaluation of her cognitive ability and possibly some form of a dementing illness.

I went to see Ms. Patricia in her hospital room at about nine in the morning. I knocked on the door and walked in. She was sitting on a chair in the corner of the room, knitting. Upon saying good morning, Ms. Patricia, to my great surprise, started laughing hysterically. My first thought was that something was wrong with my white lab coat or maybe with my hair. I excused myself and I told her I'll be right back. I went to the men's room and checked myself, but nothing was out of order, certainly nothing to explain her extreme laughter. I went back to the room, greeted her again, and this time she did not laugh.

I introduced myself as the psychiatrist covering this floor, adding that I had been asked to see her because her doctor had said she may be depressed. Ms. Patricia looked at me with surprise and straight out told me she was not depressed. I began conducting my usual psychiatric interview, asking about her past psychiatric history. She had none. She denied ever being depressed or having any symptoms of being manic, such as feeling so happy or invincible, spending money irresponsibly, being hyperactive or not sleeping enough, or behaving in an unusual sexual manner. I asked if there was a history of psychiatric problems in her family, and again she said that no members, even of her extended family, had ever had emotional problems. At one point, I reached for my notepad to write down some of what she was telling me. In doing so, I accidentally bumped into a plastic cup that was on her table. It fell to the hard floor with a loud cracking sound. Immediately Ms. Patricia began crying. *Bitterly*. I asked her why she was crying, and between sobs, she managed to tell me that she had no idea why.

45 minutes into the interview, her son walked in. I introduced myself to him and asked him to accompany me to the conference room so we could talk about his mother. The son was in his forties, well-educated and well-mannered. I asked him what he thought was going on with his mother and he indicated his complete bafflement over her condition. He said she had several relatively small strokes from which she recovered well every time, but it seemed

that her last stroke had brought on these episodes of sudden un-accountable sadness or unaccountable happiness. I asked him if there was a reason for her to feel sad and he indicated that other than having had the small strokes and having to be in the hospital, there was nothing else in her life to feel sad about. He indicated that Ms. Patricia greatly enjoyed spending time with her grandchildren.

At this point, it appeared that Ms. Patricia might be suffering from a condition called pathological laughter and crying (PLC). The strokes she had suffered would make her a prime candidate for this condition. In PLC, the connections between the higher emotional centers in the brain, where we feel happy or sad, are disconnected/severed from the lower centers that control the facial expressions of happiness or sadness. In other words, the motor programs that activate the facial features of sadness or happiness are no longer connected to the higher centers where these emotions are experienced. It seems that any stimulus, such as the door slamming or the noise of a fallen cup, could activate these lower centers and set off the motor program of crying or laughing without any input whatsoever from the higher emotional centers.

Ms. Patricia's son and I went back into the room armed with this PLC theory. Upon entering the room, I made a point of slamming the door and indeed Ms. Patricia began crying. She calmed down in a matter of seconds and we began talking about how she was feeling. I did my best to make her laugh but failed miserably. But just as I was thinking of concluding the interview and asking her son to accompany me out of the room, she burst out laughing.

It turned out that there is a simple treatment for PLC, a pill that she could take at night. As this was my first case of pathological laughter and crying, I had not tried it before. But because it was the standard treatment, I prescribed it.

Three days later I went back to visit Ms. Patricia. She was about to be discharged from the hospital. I spent 20 minutes with her during which no episodes of crying or laughing occurred. According to nursing staff, these episodes ceased to occur only 48 hours into treatment. She was indeed neither particularly sad nor happy, just very glad to be leaving the hospital.

From Pub-Med (A well-regarded source of medical knowledge and recent research findings).

Pathological laughing and crying (PLC) is a condition characterized by frequent, brief, intense paroxysms of uncontrollable crying and/or laughing due to a neurological disorder. When sufficiently frequent and severe, PLC may interfere with the performance of activities of daily living, interpersonal functioning, or both, and is a source of distress for affected patients and their families.

My Thoughts:

PLC is often misunderstood by patients and their families and is under-recognized by clinicians caring for patients with this disorder. However, this syndrome is easily recognized when understood properly and is highly responsive to treatment with a variety of pharmacological agents.

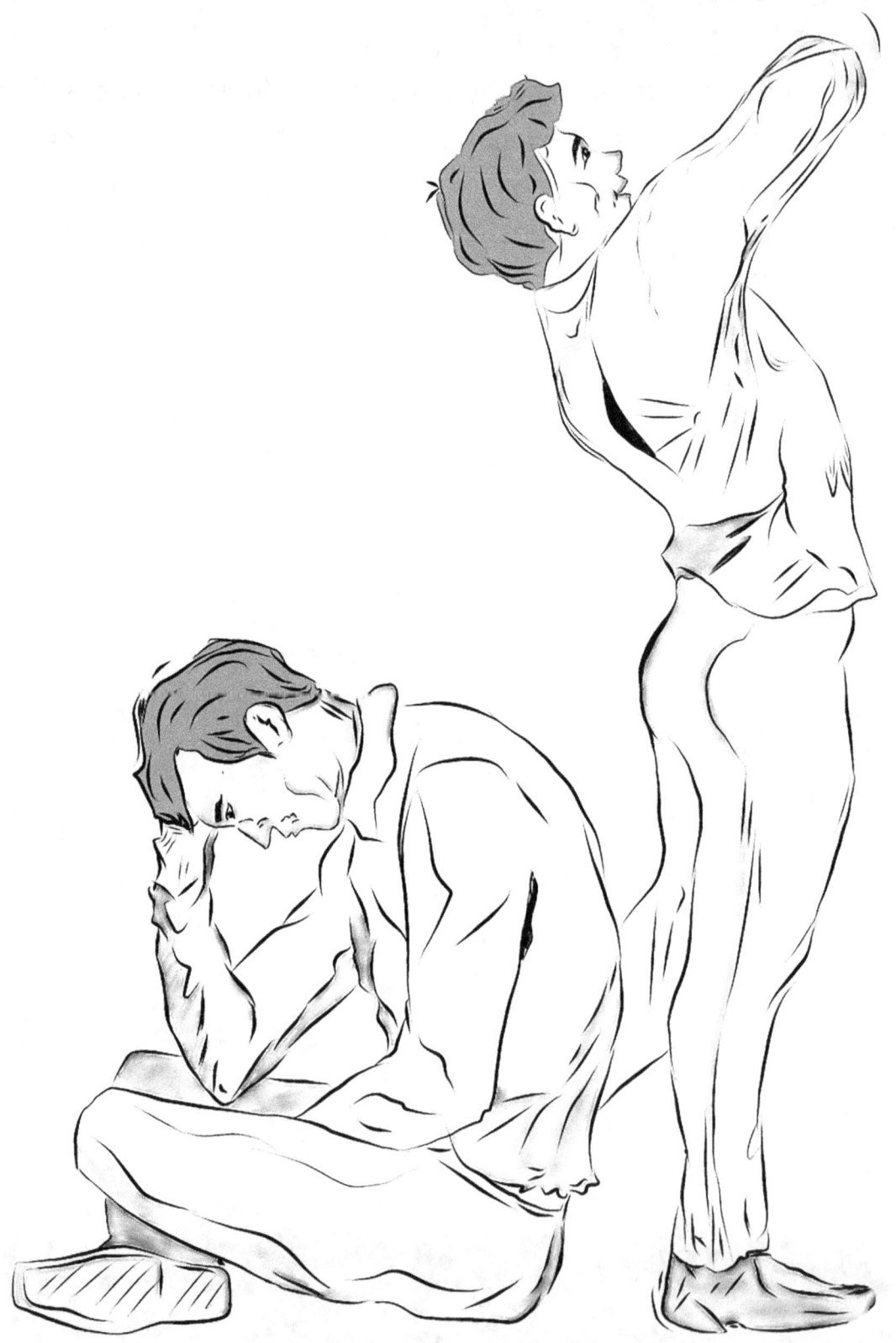

Case Four

Clozapine: A Wonder Drug for Schizophrenia

The setting for the following amazing case is an inpatient psychiatry unit in a university-run psychiatric hospital. Clark was a young man in his early thirties who had been diagnosed with schizophrenia for 14 years. He had been in many hospitals and seemed never to have complied with any treatment offered to him. He tended to escape from the hospitals but had never been violent and so did not need to be placed in secured psychiatric facilities like state-run institutions. Most recently, he had been found by the police walking on a freeway and had been brought in without resistance.

Mr. Clark was a nice young man with a high school education and two college semesters. The main features of his illness were the tendency to become paranoid and to feel that the government and his parents were after him to keep him locked up. He frequently heard voices telling him that "he was no good" and that they will "get him". He tended to set in his room and not do much. He rarely came out to watch TV and interact with staff and other patients.

Upon his admission to the present ward, which catered to patients diagnosed with schizophrenia, we [myself along with my two assigned resident trainees] reviewed his medical and psychiatric history. We immediately saw that Mr. Clark had never done well on any medications prescribed to him. Nor had he consistently taken his medications after leaving the hospital. But at this time, a new medication for treatment-resistant schizophrenia – clozapine – had just come on the market. I knew about it because one of my professors during my training had been instrumental in developing it. Mr. Clark struck me as an excellent candidate for clozapine. But one obstacle remained. The patient had no insurance, and Medicaid did not cover it. The cost at that time was about $9,000/year.

I instructed the social worker to see if there were any resources to help with this high cost. After several days of intensive search, she came back with some useful information. Mr. Clark was the son of a prominent and affluent woman in the local city government. The social worker had found her phone number.

I made the call. The mother answered and I introduced myself. I said simply that her son struck me as an ideal candidate for a promising but costly new drug. She said she did not want to hear anything about it. "Doctor," she added, "we had to let go of him. And this wound has now healed."

Naturally, I was disappointed. All I could do was start the patient on a combination of affordable medications, the best I could come up with, but I didn't have much hope. A week later, however, the social worker told me that the mother called her, wanting to talk to me. I was surprised and gladly returned her call. The first thing Ms. Clark said was "Doctor, you opened the wound and poked into it. Can you assure me that this new medicine will make a difference?" Of course, I could not be certain and told her so. I was able, however, to give her statistics documenting the effectiveness of Clozapine, hoping that she will go for it. She asked for a few days to discuss the matter with her husband and to learn more about the drug herself. With hope in my voice, I told her I would do my best to help her son.

Two days later she called back and said they were willing to pay for a trial treatment of Clozapine, but she did not want her son to know anything about it. She added that she would not visit her son at this time. "Doctor," she said, "call me back only if her son is back to normal." This was a tall order indeed, but I was glad that Ms. Clark had decided to begin the trial.

Clozapine has possible severe side effects that could lead to death. These risks required daily blood tests. Early on, Mr. Clark resisted the tests but began cooperating after several days. This was a positive sign.

A week into the treatment Mr. Clark began to speak more. He was still delusional and hearing voices, but he was now communicating better and leaving his room a bit more. By about the middle of the third week, his communication was almost normal. He was looking people in the eye and even occasionally smiling. I asked him about the voices, and he indicated that he had not heard them for the last day and a half. He was not worried about the government at this point. I was now feeling quite encouraged but I resisted the impulse to call his mother.

By the end of three weeks, he had not heard voices for five full days and had expressed no paranoid ideas. He was now out of his room most of the time and had actually made a friend on the unit. Indeed, he had improved enough to be discharged from the hospital. But knowing his prior history of non-compliance with his medications, discharging him to a group home or halfway house would likely lead to his stopping his medication and relapsing. I had no choice now but to call his mother.

I made the phone call and described Mr. Clark's progress. Ms. Clark heard this news in tears. I asked if she would be willing to come to visit her son and help us with the discharge planning. She agreed, and the next morning she arrived with her husband. While not the patient's biological father, he knew Mr. Clark well. It was an emotional reunion. Mr. Clark threw himself into his mother's embrace upon seeing her. The meeting went on for 40 minutes. In the end, the mother looked at me and asked if she could take him home. I could not have been happier.

DSM-5 Diagnostic Criteria for Schizophrenia

*Two (or more) of the following, each present for a significant portion of time during a 1-month period (or less if successfully treated). At least one of these must be delusions, hallucinations, or disorganized speech:

- Delusions
- Hallucinations
- Disorganized speech (e.g., frequent derailment or incoherence)
- Grossly disorganized or catatonic behavior
- Negative symptoms (i.e., diminished emotional expression or avolition)

* Continuous signs of the disturbance persist for at least 6 months.

*For a significant portion of time since the onset of the disturbance, the level of functioning in one or more major areas, such as work, interpersonal relations, or self-care is markedly below the level achieved prior to the onset (or when the onset is in childhood or adolescence, there is a failure to achieve expected level of interpersonal, academic, or occupational functioning).

*Schizoaffective disorder and depressive or bipolar disorder with psychotic features have been ruled out.

*The disturbance is not attributable to the physiological effects of a substance (e.g., a drug of abuse, a medication) or another medical condition.

*If there is a history of autism spectrum disorder or a communication disorder of childhood onset, the additional diagnosis of schizophrenia is made only if prominent delusions or hallucinations, in addition to the other required symptoms of schizophrenia, are also present for at least 1 month (or less if successfully treated).

My Thoughts:

If I had any doubts regarding the nature of schizophrenia being a brain disorder before I cared for Mr. Clark, I had absolutely none afterward. His recovery was nothing short of miraculous. In my experience and those of many of my colleagues, the likelihood that this improvement would continue long-term was highly probable as long as the patient continued the treatment.

I recall, visiting the professor who had helped develop this medication a few years later. He invited me and my wife to an outing at which he had invited all his patients who were on Clozapine along with their families. It was a remarkable experience. Neither my wife nor I (and I'm an expert) could tell who was a "patient" and who was a "family member". Clozapine was that effective. And today, not only that the cost of clozapine has significantly been reduced, but the medication is also now covered by all insurance including Medicaid.

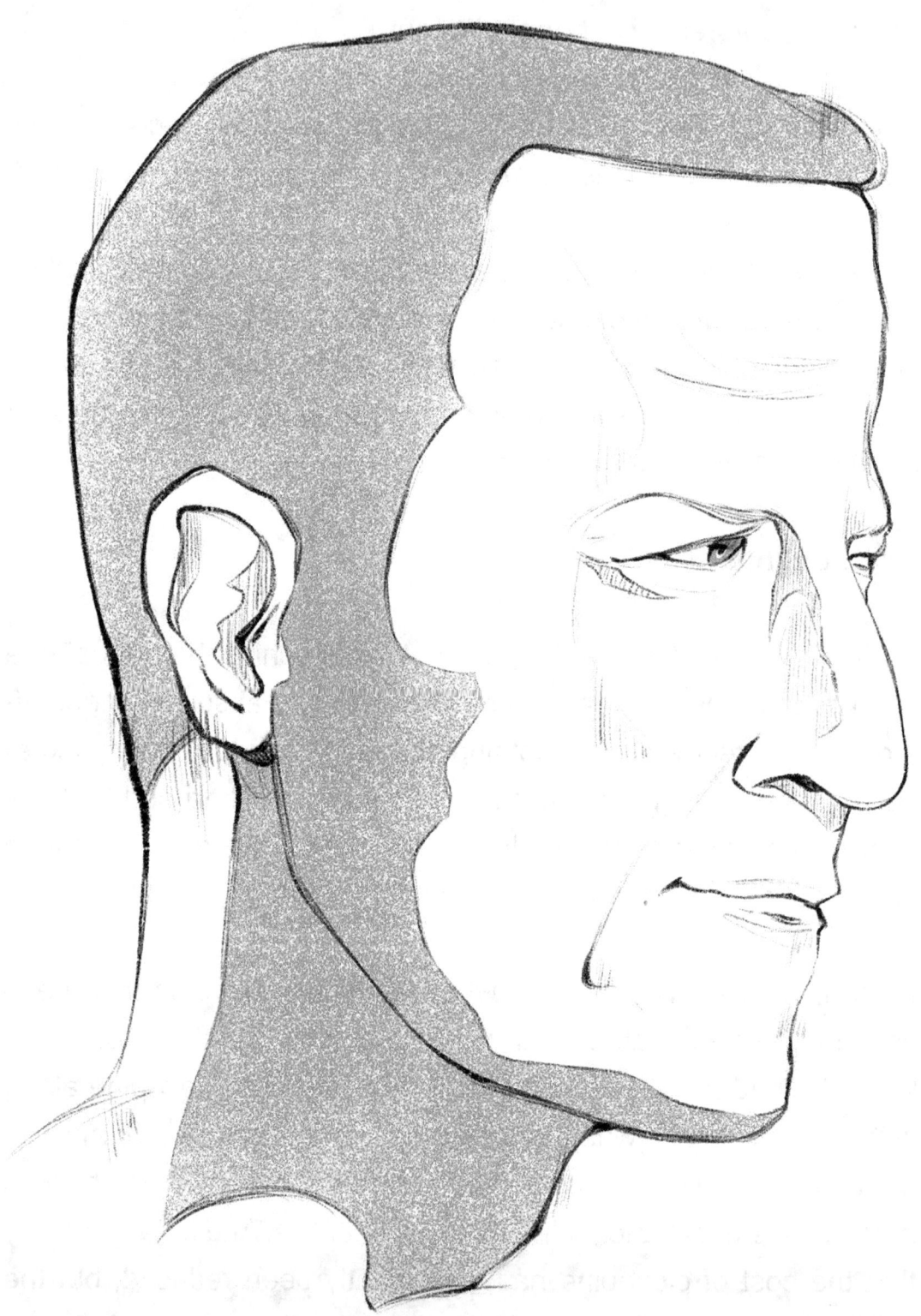

Case Five

Schizophrenia? I think not!

In Psychiatry Research Units ongoing studies are usually conducted by one or more investigators. Many of the resulting research studies are the final stages for pharmaceutical medications that will be released for clinical use pending a successful final test. At the time of this case, I was one of the research investigators on a unit in a university-run psychiatric institution. The unit was fully staffed, including a social worker stationed full-time at the institution's triage/emergency unit. Her job was simply to scout incoming patients as possibly suitable candidates for the various ongoing research studies of the Research Unit.

One morning the police brought in a 32-year-old male whom they had found wandering the streets of the city. He was disheveled and looked confused and agitated. During the entry interview, the patient was able to orient himself as to who he was and where he was in the hospital. Asked why he was wandering in the streets, his only answer was, "Anywhere I go, they find me." The social worker then asked him if he had ever participated in research involving new medications; he said no. Would he now be willing to consider being part of a research study of a new medication? He inquired about details of the study quite sensibly, asking also what might be in it for him.

The social worker gave him all the appropriate information. She told him the study would entail a thorough workup for an accurate diagnosis of his condition, based on state-of-the-art diagnostic tools.

He would then undergo a one-week period of being washed out of all medications currently in his system. The social worker also assured him that if his condition were to worsen while off all medications, he will promptly receive all appropriate medications and needed treatment. The patient, Mr. Amad, thought all this over for perhaps 30 seconds, turned to the social worker, and pointedly asked her if he had heard correctly when she said she would take him off *all* medications. She nodded affirmatively and again explained that after his system was empty of all medications, he would blindly and randomly be assigned to either the passive or active cohort of this research study. If assigned to the passive cohort, his medication would be an inactive form of medication: a placebo. If assigned to the active cohort, his medication would be the one being tested. Researchers, she emphasized, deemed it superior to any medication currently available. He was also assured that he would be closely observed at all times for any ill effects of the new medication. And if any were observed, he will be tended to immediately at no cost. Finally, he was assured of his right to withdraw from the study at any time.

Mr. Amad nodded his agreement, and a consent form was provided for him, and the social worker reviewed it with him in detail to ensure he understood what he was getting into. To her surprise, he seemed to understand her completely; his questions about the process were numerous and appropriate. He looked glad to sign the consent form and to be part of the study. He was then transferred to a room at the Research Unit.

I went to interview Mr. Amad after reviewing the information provided by the triage department (including the police report) and the social worker. His records indicated a case of chronic paranoid schizophrenia coupled with a history of non-compliance with his medications. Mr. Amad had in addition a history of anger outbursts and threatening behavior, though no evidence of having harmed anyone.

At first, I found him less than communicative. As we spoke, he looked away, as if at a distance. Apart from anger, I could initially elicit no emotions even while trying to establish friendly contact. I asked the routine questions relating to a diagnosis of schizophrenia, including whether he had been hearing voices. This he emphatically denied. When I asked if he thought there was a conspiracy against him, he answered that his parents were in cahoots with the police to find him whenever he escaped from psychiatric institutions. When they did, they would bring him back to "shoot him up" with medications he hated. At this point, he volunteered that the main reason he had volunteered to participate in this research study was the news that he would be taken off all medications and never forced to take any medications against his will.

I now felt I had enough information to feel comfortable with the diagnosis as schizophrenic. I accepted him into the research study, as I was authorized to do. The next morning, I reviewed his overnight nursing notes before visiting with him a second time. These notes indicated a few anger outbursts which had been interpreted as responding to hearing voices (the usual nursing term used is "responding to internal stimuli".) With these voices in mind, I asked Mr. Amad about last night and what might have caused his outbursts. He looked me square in the eye and said, "Here I am, sir, locked up for no good reason. Wouldn't you be angry if you were in my shoes?" Intrigued but not fully satisfied with this answer, I asked him if he had heard voices at the times of last night's anger outbursts? His answer was emphatic: "I already told you that I have never heard voices in my entire life." Now he was upset indeed!

Well, having frequently heard exactly those responses from demonstrably schizophrenia patients in the past, I did not take Mr. Amad's denial too seriously. He was now on his second day of the one-week medication washout. During the evening, he was again offered calming medications, but this time he declined them with no trace of anger. The nurses said he was now cooperative, and the staff did not feel it was necessary to force the calming medications. He was not threatening himself or anyone else.

It was now day three of the washout period. I visited him again, this time to try to gauge the severity of his psychotic symptoms (i.e., the voices and the paranoid feelings). Once again, he denied hearing voices. I explained the concept of hallucination. He said he understood it but had never experienced hallucinations. He now sounded more credible to me, showing more affect and presence of mind. His face was more animated. He smiled occasionally and even asked me how *I* was doing. He seemed to be doing better *off* medications than *on*. I was puzzled.

Day four of the washout came without the patient having exhibited any clear psychotic symptoms whatsoever. Anger outbursts were now infrequent. But now I was in a dilemma. If I could not verify his psychotic symptoms, he will not meet the required criteria for admission to the research study! So, I grabbed a cup of coffee for an extended discussion with Mr. Amad. We spoke comfortably but found him loathe to divulge details of his life. We finished our coffee, and I shook hands with him, all of which felt normal. My puzzlement was growing. I was now close to concluding that he did not meet the criteria for the research study.

It was the weekend, so I did not see Mr. Amad for two days as he continued his washout period. Monday morning was the seventh and final day of the washout. He topped my to-do list now as I had to make a final decision about his participation in the study. I went to talk to him, coffee in hand. He had just finished breakfast and was drinking coffee (only decaf was served on the unit). As I approached him, he smiled and reached out to shake hands. He looked normal, and our interaction felt normal. I grabbed a chair and sat down. I started by telling him frankly that as of this moment he no longer met the criteria for the research study, and I really wanted to know what his story was.

That did it! To my amazement, he finally opened up. At age 13 he had been a poor student, having difficulty with all his classes, being unable to sit still in class, and falling hopelessly behind. His friends were all like him with similar classroom attention and performance issues. They liked to cut school and head into town for marijuana. His parents had found him out and, thinking something was seriously wrong with him, brought him to a psychiatrist. According to Mr. Amad the psychiatrist spent less than 15 minutes with him. That's all it took for this professional to inform his parents that their son suffered from schizophrenia and required instant hospitalization. "So, they forced me into a psychiatric ward. What a horrible experience. When I refused their medications, they would tie me down and stick needles into me. Injections. Injections that took away my soul. I hated every minute of it. I hate psychiatrists now. They all are full of baloney."

Oh my God, I thought to myself. Could it be true that all that this patient was suffering from was attention deficit hyperactivity disorder (ADHD)? Had his life been ruined by a hasty diagnosis? It struck me that there exists a respected and standard rating scale for the diagnosis of ADHD. But then it hit me that there exist no objective laboratory tests to diagnose the condition of schizophrenia, as is the case for all psychiatric disorders, as of 2022 (see My Thoughts below). I promptly administered Mr. Amad the standardized ADHD rating scale. It assessed both his current symptoms and his symptoms as a child. He fully met the ADHD criteria for both periods. There was no room for doubt.

I promptly started Mr. Amad on ADHD medication. Immediately he felt more relaxed and connected. I then had to tell him the bad news and the good news: he was no longer part of the research study, but he was not suffering from schizophrenia! I apologized to him on behalf of the field of psychiatry and sent him to an appropriate housing facility selected by the social worker, who herself was as amazed as I was at the outcome of Mr. Amad's case.

DSM-5 Criteria for ADHD in an adult

All criteria must be met for a diagnosis of ADHD in adults:

- Five or more symptoms of inattention and/or ≥5 symptoms of hyperactivity/impulsivity must have persisted for ≥6 months to a degree that is inconsistent with the developmental level and negatively impacts social and academic/occupational activities.

- Several symptoms (inattentive or hyperactive/impulsive) were present before the age of 12 years.
- Several symptoms (inattentive or hyperactive/impulsive) must be present in ≥2 settings (e.g., at home, school, or work; with friends or relatives; in other activities).
- There is clear evidence that the symptoms interfere with or re-duce the quality of social, academic, or occupational functioning.
- Symptoms do not occur exclusively during schizophrenia or another psychotic disorder and are not better explained by another mental disorder (e.g., mood disorder, anxiety dis-order, dissociative disorder, personality disorder, substance intoxication, or withdrawal).

My Thoughts:

My time with Mr. Amad showed me just how crucial a patient's first encounter with psychiatry can be. First impressions can mean ev-erything! Earning or losing the trust of a patient (and family) is half the battle at least. The first hour (or even 15 minutes!) can shape a lifelong attitude toward the field. I decided not to trust a diagnosis passed on to me unless I knew and trusted the clinician making it. Even then, I decided that a full and thorough work-up should ac-company that first encounter.

As mentioned above, while there are no laboratory-based objective tests for any psychiatric disorder, there are well-standardized rating scales. These are comprised of standardized questions that can be administered by a clinician or self-administered by the patient. Most certainly, adding such scales to the clinical interview improves diagnostic accuracy, but such scales still heavily depend on the responses given by the patient or the impressions of the family. The accuracy of objective laboratory tests, on the other hand, would not hinge on the cooperativeness of the patient or their accurate perception of their symptoms.

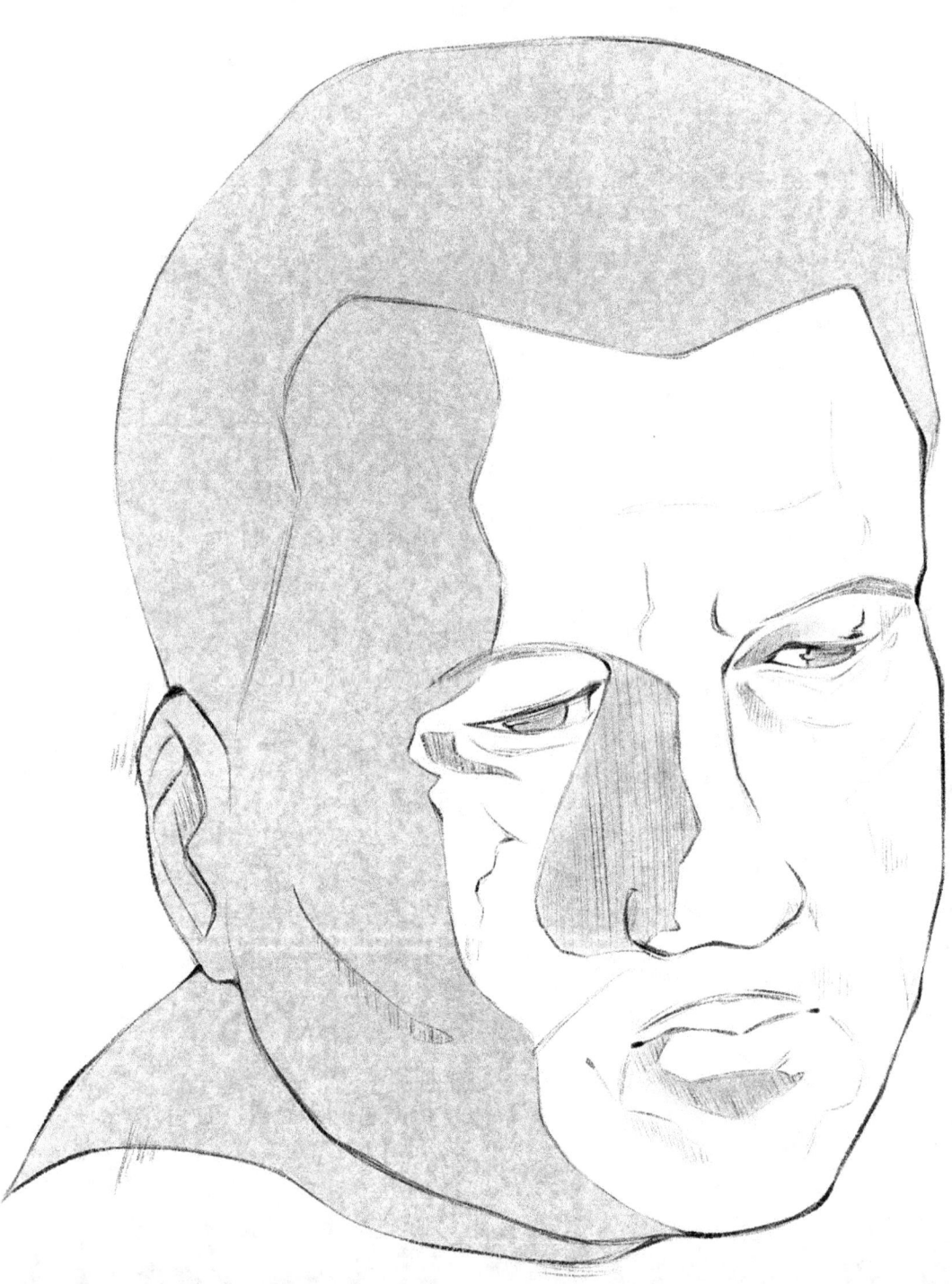

Case Six

Did He Have Schizophrenia or Not?
And Did It Really Matter?

While serving on an inpatient service unit of a university-affiliated county hospital, I saw many patients diagnosed with schizophrenia. The case, of Mr. David, was instructive to me regarding the status of the system of care for the mentally ill in the US.

Mr. David, as I'll call him, was in his early forties, single, and living in a group home for the mentally ill. Mr. David had not been employed for the last 20 years and was receiving Social Security Disability payments. He had no friendships or social relationships except for minimal interactions with staff and residents at his group home. He had a long history of brief hospitalizations triggered every time by a flare-up of his psychotic symptoms. Each hospital's routine was to reevaluate his medications and to make adjustments to bring his symptoms under control. He was then discharged to the group home. This routine usually took about a week.

My standard approach and my teaching to medical students and Psychiatry residents is that the clinician should not simply accept prior assessments as accurate. This is of course unless one knows the prior clinician and has a high level of confidence and regard for them. Otherwise, the patient should be re-evaluated to assess the veracity of the diagnosis and the prescribed management plan.

As I began this process, I realized that there were several problems including a history of repeated head injuries resulting from fights as a youngster compounded by a history of a supposed minor stroke that was shortly followed by the onset of Mr. David's psychiatric symptoms. Furthermore, upon assessment of the psychiatric symptoms exhibited by Mr. David, his psychotic symptoms were absolutely limited to his belief that all his misfortunes in life were caused by some agency that was somehow related to the government and out to destroy him. Although he had no further details about this agency, his belief in this conspiracy was fixed and unshakeable. I could find no other psychotic symptoms in him, including hallucination in any form. Mr. David simply did not meet the criteria for a diagnosis of paranoid schizophrenia. Instead, he was most likely suffering from a Delusional Disorder that causes patients to cling to a delusional and encapsulated belief in a non-bizarre [i.e., could possibly happen as compared to bizarre ideas like being invaded by Marchant's or being completely hollowed from the inside] idea. In other words, his delusional system was limited to a single false belief and was accompanied by no other psychotic symptoms.

Given Mr. David's history of diagnosed brain injuries and a questionable minor stroke, I wondered whether they might relate to his psychiatric symptoms. So, we began an organic work-up, as it's commonly called. This involved two tests: magnetic resonance imaging (MRI) and an electroencephalograph (EEG). Where the MRI would show structural problems with Mr. David's brain, the EEG would assess its overall functionality. It's worth noting that results of both tests for schizophrenia patients tend to fall within the norms of results for healthy individuals.

For Mr. David, both tests proved to be abnormal, indicating significant damage to the brain structure and function. Given the chronology between when the brain injuries occurred and the emergence of the psychotic symptoms, I felt comfortable changing the diagnosis from Chronic Paranoid Schizophrenia (CPD) to Organic Delusional Disorder (ODD). I felt confident that I had corrected a major diagnostic error. Mr. David could pursue his life knowing that he was not suffering from a genetic and heritable disorder (schizophrenia) but from an organic and non-heritable one (ODD).

Medication adjustment went as planned and the patient understood his new diagnosis and was happy to have finally shed off the diagnosis of schizophrenia. He was subsequently discharged back to the group home.

At this point, I received one of the major professional awakenings of my career. Two weeks passed and the social worker came running to inform me that because I had rejected the diagnosis of schizophrenia the patient was no longer qualified to receive disability payments. My diligent diagnostic work had thus created a huge financial problem for Mr. David. Worse yet, the disability office had told the social worker they hadn't even heard of the new diagnosis of organic delusional disorder. Only schizophrenia was on their books. So, Mr. David would have to leave his group home. The social worker begged me to reconsider my diagnosis and very reluctantly I felt obligated to comply.

In the battle between insurance and medicine, insurance had won.

PubMed: Organic Delusional Disorder.

A mental disorder caused by intrinsic brain disease which is characterized by persistent or recurrent irrational beliefs. Consciousness and memory are not affected. It may be broadly classified as a psychotic disorder due to a general medical condition.

Organic psychoses are believed to result from a physical defect of or damage to the brain. Functional psychoses are believed to have no physical brain disease evident upon clinical examination. That is not to say that there is no biological abnormality as the bases of the disorder but as of now laboratory tests including brain imaging that can diagnose the disorder are yet to be developed.

My Thoughts:

While the DSM-5 book lists more than 220 psychiatric diagnoses, only a few [less than ten] are considered "Severe and Persistent". The benefit payments to which a patient is entitled are based on the classification of the disorder. In my experience, not some but all psychiatric disorders not only cause suffering but greatly impair social and economic productivity. In my experience, "Severe and Persistent," as presently determined, is highly arbitrary and most of the time is simply harmful to patients.

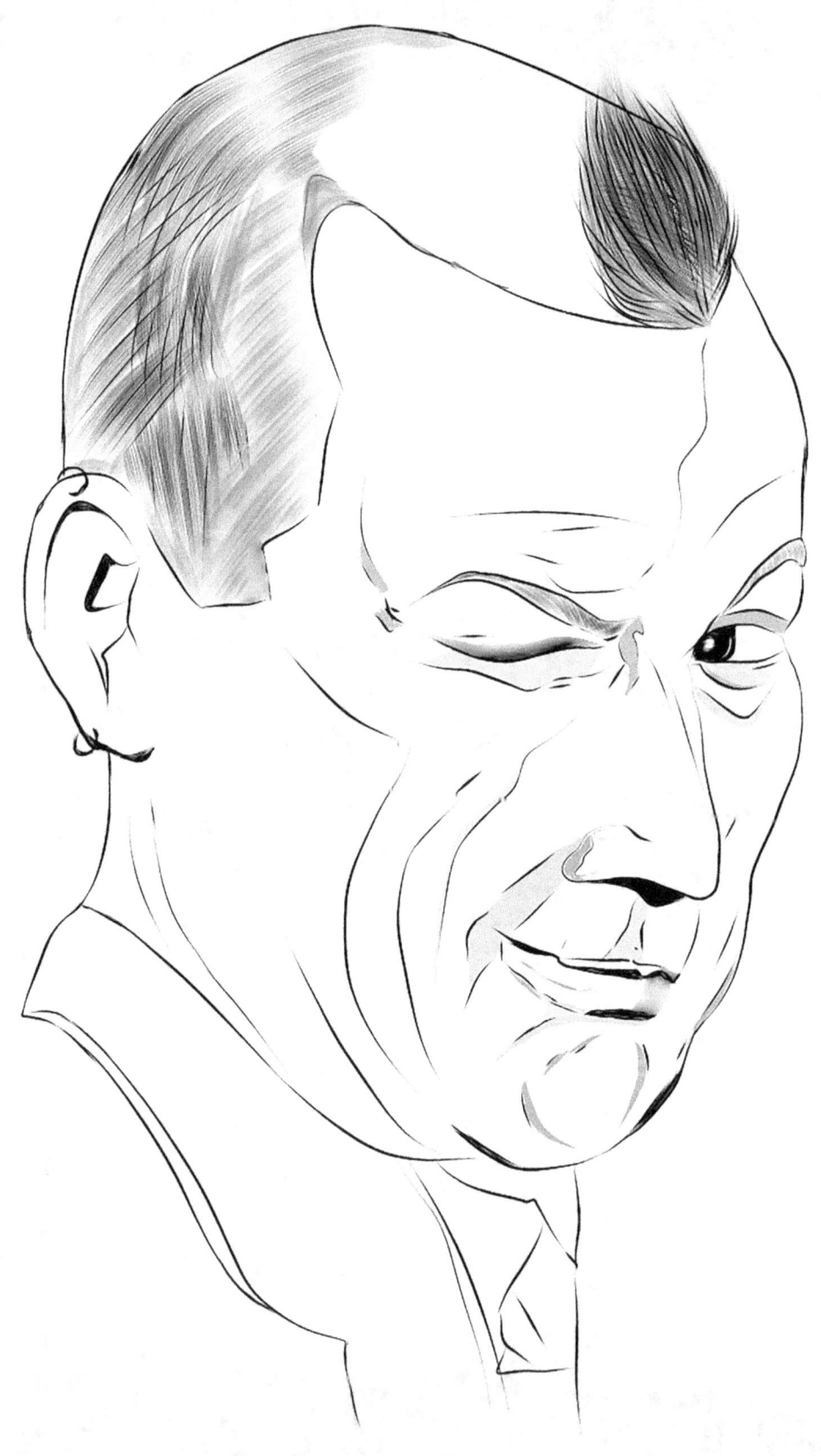

Case Seven

A Schizophrenic or a Con Artist?
The Patient Who Fooled Me!

Mr. Frank was admitted to an adult psychiatry inpatient unit after he became extremely rowdy and aggressive in a bar. When the police arrived, they found him incoherent, confused, and agitated. Upon arrival at the emergency room at the hospital, he was noticed to be responding to auditory hallucinations (imaginary voices). He was talking to several imaginary people. The hospital had no prior records for him. He was given calming medications and sent up to the unit.

After a full nursing assessment in the unit, it was soon agreed that Mr. Frank was suffering from schizophrenia, with the main symptom of auditory hallucinations. The psychiatry resident assigned to the unit saw him the same day and fully concurred with this assessment. I first saw Mr. Frank the next morning. One hallmark of schizophrenia is abnormal eye contact. But far from just avoiding eye contact, it was as if Mr. Frank was looking not away from me but straight *through* me. A most uncomfortable feeling! Over the years I would come to regard such behavior as useful in diagnosing schizophrenia. Based on all the information available and examining Mr. Frank, I too confirmed the diagnosis of schizophrenia and started Mr. Frank on an appropriate course of treatment with antipsychotic medication.

As the days passed, the patient improved slowly. He reported the voices to be less loud and less frequent. But still bothersome. On day five the team began discussing discharge planning. But Mr. Frank had no place to go. The social worker started planning to place him in a halfway house, a therapeutic setting maintained by the state. Here social workers call on residents to ensure their steady compliance with recommended treatments and follow-up appointments. The process of placing a patient into a halfway-house system would require several days and the social worker began the paperwork.

Now we were on day eight with Mr. Frank having significantly improved in many aspects except for his highly unusual and off-putting eye contact. I saw him that morning and approved his discharge pending completion of the halfway house arrangements by the social worker. As it happened, my office was located just outside the door to the inpatient unit. I had finished my morning rounds and was walking to my office to work on a scientific paper about schizophrenia for submission to a major international journal. And there standing outside my office door were three police officers. One asked if I knew where Mr. Frank was. I said I did. And, that he was my patient. I introduced myself and asked if there was any problem.

The officer informed me that they had a warrant for Mr. Frank's arrest. I was taken aback. I stated with some protest in my voice "He came to us with a bad episode of schizophrenia. And he has just started to get better". "Schizophrenic, my ass," objected the officer. "We know this man well. He's a fox. Acting crazy is his modus operandi for avoiding us after he's done something bad. This time its robbery". After satisfying myself that the officers had cause for an arrest, I gave them my OK for the arrest. But I still believed Mr. Frank suffered from schizophrenia. All I could do was to comfort myself with the thought that at a minimum we had brought his disability under some control, and he could at least continue to take his medications while in prison.

Soon the officers had Mr. Frank in handcuffs. As they were passing my office, my former patient peeked inside, looked me right in the eye, for the first time, and to my astonishment declared, "It's been fun, Doc!"

The officers had been correct. Mr. Frank did not have schizophrenia. A con artist has taken me in. This is despite my years of experience with schizophrenia patients. What struck me now was the absence of *objective* biological diagnostic tests for any of the over 200 different psychiatric disorders we currently know of. Only the careful observations of neuroscience could provide them. These tests would be a crucial step if the field of psychiatry was ever going to free itself from the stigma of frequent misdiagnosis of which my own misdiagnosis of Mr. Frank was a painful example.

My Thoughts:

As of 2022, the field of Psychiatry has yet to develop even one biological-objective test that can confidently tell a patient from a non-patient. That said, I have spent much of my research career in somewhat frustrating attempts to develop data-based biological diagnostic tests as well as providing guidance for developing such tests. Tests that would greatly reduce errors stemming from the subjective psychiatric evaluations that are the current standard in the field.

In non-psychiatric fields, the use of data-based laboratory tests to validate preliminary subjective diagnoses has become standard. These tests evaluate the status of virtually all non-psychiatric disorders. As a screener [early and non-definitive tests when a condition is suspected], the tests would be administered to patients requiring more detailed assessment for a definitive diagnosis. The absence of these tests in the field of psychiatry cannot be attributed to a scarcity of candidates. Biological research into the pathophysiology of psychiatric disorders has yielded many highly replicable abnormalities with abundant potential for development into clinically useful laboratory tests.

Research into the readiness for biological abnormalities to be tested diagnostically has produced a large body of literature documenting the existence of recordable abnormalities in certain patient populations as compared to normal controls. This is encouraging. But on the other hand, the literature describing the steps required for the creation of clinic-ready tests for these abnormalities is scant indeed.

The development of clinic-ready diagnostic procedures is critical if ever the field of psychiatry will get past the stigma caused by the crisis of diagnostic obscurity and error that has impaired its effectiveness from its earliest days.

This is no exaggeration. Consider the large field of forensic psychiatry. And take a murder case, one where the accused faces the death penalty. The defense, while acknowledging physical guilt, has contended that the accused suffers from a mental disorder that contributed to his committing the crime. The prosecution wants nothing of this argument. So how can it be resolved? Psychiatry has no clear answer; indeed, it plays both sides of the game. Dueling (but of course highly qualified) forensic psychiatrists take the stand in the service of prosecution and defense. And if that isn't enough, the arbiters of their conflicting testimony are twelve laypersons unfamiliar or ignorant of psychiatric practice.

Consider now how the existence of objective diagnostic tests could serve the interests of justice better than they are served now.

In an earlier book, I made a proposal regarding the situation when a laboratory-based biological variable has been observed to be deviant from healthy controls in a given patient population. I proposed that the scientific community take note and spare no expense in determining whether this deviation is suitable for diagnostic purposes. We devised four steps towards this goal in *Humanist Psychiatry*, 2nd Edition (Boutros NN, 2022).

Reference:

Boutros, Nash N. *Humanist Psychiatry*, 2nd Edition. NOVA Science Publishers, New York, NY, 2022.

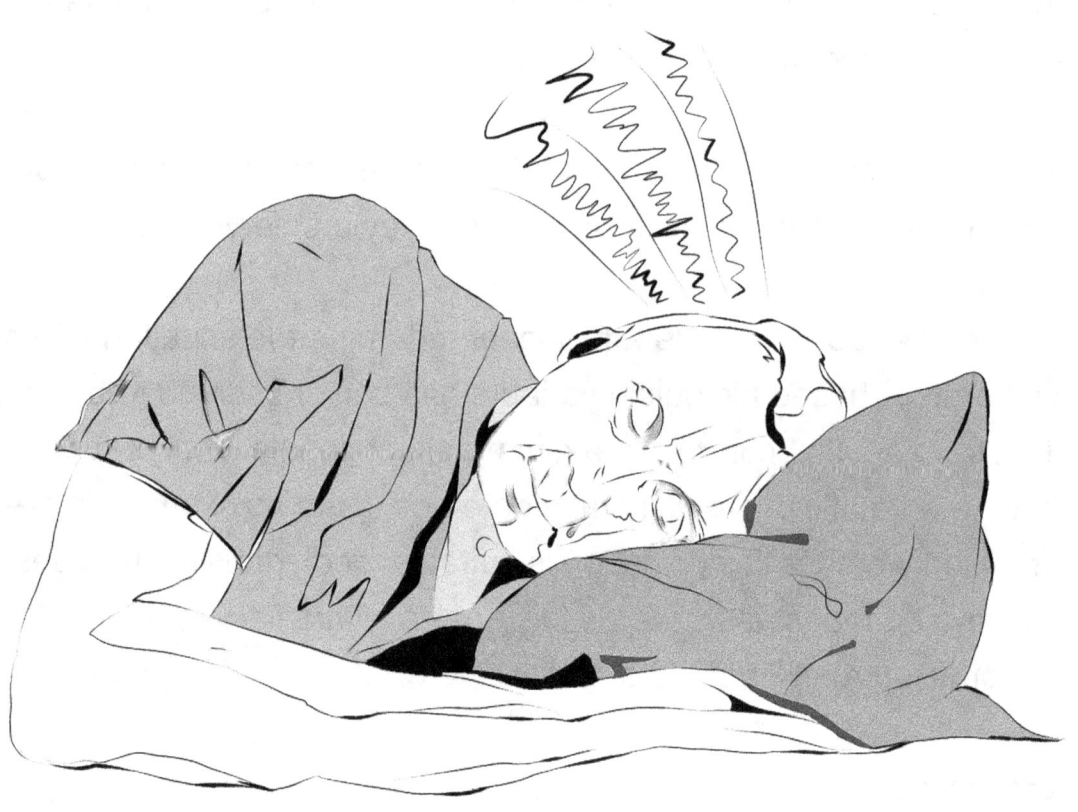

Case Eight

The Convincing Power of Science

As with Ms. Patricia in case number three, I was holding a dual appointment in the departments of Psychiatry and Neurology at a major university hospital. This combination enabled me to successfully manage the condition of one Mr. Raoul. He was a 64-year-old business executive, highly successful by all accounts, and with a stable home and social life. But Mr. Raoul had recently begun missing important deadlines, showing up late to work, and frequently unshaven. Noting these changes, his colleagues at work, including his supervising manager tried to help him, but he flat-out denied any problems. As Mr. Raoul's condition deteriorated, his boss felt compelled to ask him to go see a doctor. After a discussion with his wife, Mr. Raoul saw his general practitioner, who tentatively concluded Mr. Raoul was suffering from depression and then ordered a full battery of lab tests to obtain an accurate diagnosis.

All test results came back within normal ranges, a result that was not inconsistent with depression. So, Mr. Raoul's doctor advised him to see a psychiatrist to discuss his apparent depression. But this suggestion, made in the presence of Mr. Raoul and his wife, enraged him. He accused his physician of incompetence and stormed out of his office, his wife in hand.

Happily, the doctor didn't throw in the towel. Instead, called the chairperson of the Department of Neurology at the University

Hospital. What options were open to him, he wanted to know, for a patient likely suffering from depression who flatly refused to see a psychiatrist? One promising option, he was told, was the availability of a physician who was doubly trained as a psychiatrist and a neurologist. He led a clinic housed in the hospital's neurology department. He had me in mind. Mr. Raoul's internist proceeded to contact Mr. Raoul, saying he had good news, and he could meet with a physician at the department of Neurology. He gave my name, conveniently omitting that I was a psychiatrist as well.

I reviewed the records received from his internist, and I fully concurred that Mr. Raoul was probably suffering from Major Depressive Disorder (MDD). At the appointment, Mr. Raoul appeared on time with his wife. I made a point to wear my white lab coat (as I did even when I was seeing patients in the Psychiatry Clinic). I conducted a full medical and neurological examination on the patient, including asking some questions relating to signs and symptoms of depression without using that word.

As an expert in the field of brain waves (Electroencephalography or EEG) and its clinical applications in psychiatric settings, I was aware that MDD has signature abnormalities in the sleep of patients. Specifically, the stages of sleep known as rapid eye movement (REM sleep) tend to appear earlier in the night in a symptom known as early-REM-onset. Furthermore, and still more specifically for depression, the intensity of the rapid eye movements increases significantly to the extent that researchers sometimes call them

REM storms. But these sleep changes do not occur in every single case of MDD and so themselves do not confirm a diagnosis of MDD. Nonetheless, the presence of these sleep abnormalities is a strong indicator of MDD. For the sake of this patient, I was hoping that he would exhibit these changes in his sleep recording. With this hope in mind, I ordered an overnight sleep study.

Mr. Raoul had no objection to the sleep test after I explained the strong relationship that exists between a good night's sleep and one's overall feeling of well-being. He appeared on time for the study, and it went smoothly. I got the results within 36 hours and was relieved to see that my patient did indeed exhibit both sleep changes indicative of MDD.

Mr. Raoul saw me the following Monday and he came, as before, with his wife. I started by showing him what a normal sleep recording looks like, explaining to him that normal sleep includes four to five sleep cycles beginning with falling into light sleep (stages one and two) and then falling into progressively deeper stages of sleep (stages three and four) prior to arriving at the first REM cycle some 80-90 minutes after falling asleep. This cycle repeats four to five times nightly, usually in a smooth fashion that shows up as a clear pattern on the sleep recording chart.

Next, we compared his recording with the normal one. He immediately saw the difference. I carefully explained to him the nature of the abnormalities in his recording, pointing to the chart showing the first REM cycle coming much earlier than normal noting the unusual density of his REM periods. He looked at me and asked what could cause such changes. That was the question I was hoping for. "It's called Major Depressive Disorder.," I said. He thought for a minute. "Depression," he said hesitantly, "isn't that a *psychological* disorder? How on earth can you record a brain abnormality caused by a merely *psychological* problem?" The wonderment behind this question gave me the opening to tell Mr. Raoul about the biochemical changes that neuroscience has found are *invariably* associated with MDD. He was all ears now. When I stopped talking, he paused, looked at me, and asked the humblest of questions: was anything that can be done about it?

My patient was now open to hearing about medications that work overtime to correct the biochemical abnormalities associated with MDD. These I discussed with him, along with their effectiveness, side effects, and a fairly impressive record of success. Mr. Raoul seemed ready to proceed with them, but I could tell that thoughts were still whirling around in his head. I gave him all the time he needed to mull over this revelation and to make a final decision about treatment. It didn't take long. In a few seconds, he looked at me again and said he was willing to give it a try. I then prescribed an antidepressant medication that I had success with and hoping for the best. He agreed to return for a checkup in two weeks, or any time sooner if needed.

He returned in two weeks with his wife, and they both agreed that at a minimum he was sleeping better and showing up to work on time more often. I took this as an indication that maybe the medication was beginning to work, and we set his next appointment in three weeks.

When he walked into my office this time, he was cheerful, clean-shaven, and had energy in his step. He did not bring his wife. He was back to work, fully functioning. He made it clear that taking a scientific route in addressing his condition is what had caused him to accept treatment. He stated emphatically that he believes in science.

DSM-5 Major Depressive Disorder (MDD)

Depressive symptoms

- ≥5 symptoms during the same two-week period that are a change from previous functioning; depressed mood and/or loss of interest/pleasure must be present; exclude symptoms clearly attributable to another medical condition
- Depressed mood most of the day, nearly every day; maybe subjective (e.g., feels sad, empty, hopeless) or observed by others (e.g., appears tearful); in children and adolescents, can be irritable mood
- Loss of interest/pleasure. Markedly diminished interest/pleasure in all (or almost all) activities most of the day, nearly every day; maybe subjective or observed by other
- Weight loss or gain. Significant weight loss (without dieting) or gain (change of >5% body weight in a month) or decrease or increase in appetite nearly every day; in children, may be a failure to gain weight as expected.

- Insomnia or hypersomnia nearly every day.
- Psychomotor agitation or retardation nearly every day and observable by others (not merely subjectively restless or slow).
- Fatigue or loss of energy, nearly every day.
- Feeling worthless or excessive/inappropriate guilt nearly every day; guilt may be delusional; not merely self-reproach or guilt about being sick.
- Decreased concentration nearly every day; maybe indecisiveness; may be subjective or observed by others
- Thoughts of death/suicide. Recurrent thoughts of death (not just fear of dying), recurrent suicidal ideation without a specific plan, or suicide attempt, or a specific plan for suicide

Additional required criteria:

- Symptoms cause clinically significant distress or impairment in social, occupational, or other important areas of functioning.
- Episode not attributable to physiological effects of a substance or another medical condition.
- Episode not better explained by schizoaffective disorder, schizophrenia, schizophreniform disorder, delusional disorder, or other specified and unspecified schizophrenia spectrum and other psychotic disorders.
- No history of a manic or hypomanic episode.
- Exclusion does not apply if all manic-like or hypomanic-like episodes are substance-induced or are attributable to physiological effects of another medical condition.

My Thoughts:

As I have already indicated, it is my firm belief that the next major evolution in the field of psychiatry will be the development of reliable biological diagnostic tests for all psychiatric disorders. Such tests may not be limited to diagnosis but may also predict likely responses to treatment. I'm happy to say that the evidence that such tests will be available in the fairly near future is rapidly accumulating.

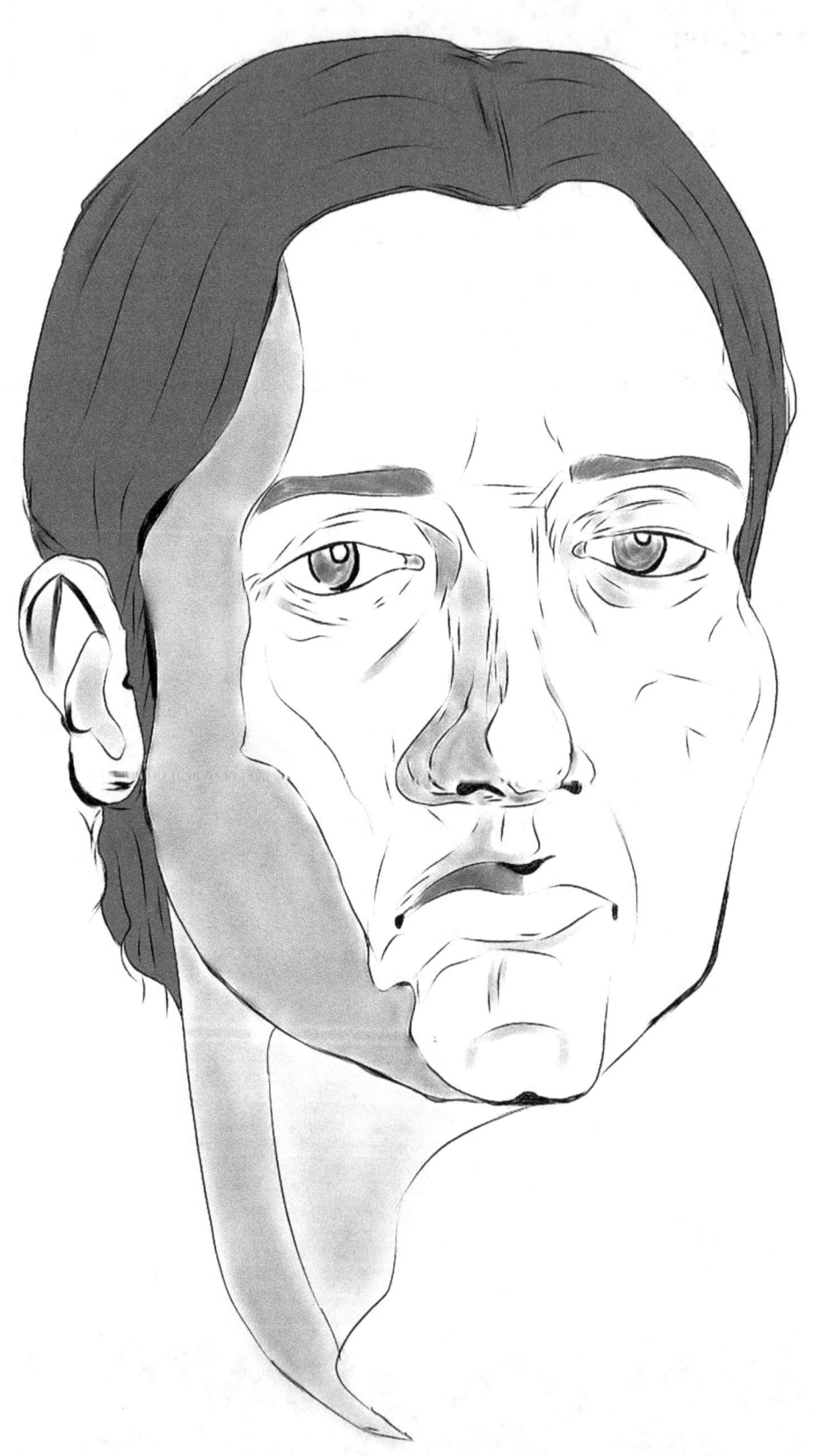

Case Nine

The Borderline Woman I Could Not Help

Borderline Personality Disorder (BPD) is one of the most intriguing and subtle of psychiatric disorders, and, as exemplified in Case One, is also the disorder that drew me to the field of psychiatric clinical research. Here is a second BPD case that defied not only my expertise but also that of my colleagues at a nationally recognized academic psychiatric center.

Barbara was a 26-year-old female, twice divorced, who was going through her life with a diagnosis of BPD. She had been referred to me when her respected psychiatrist, whom she has seen for about a year, retired and it was my turn to take the next referral from his caseload. This was a university-affiliated general psychiatry practice.

I reviewed all notes and records received from her previous therapist. Two things stood out. First, she had been accurately diagnosed with BPD. Second, she was not responding to any form of treatment, be it medication or psychotherapy. As is the case with most practicing psychiatrists, the focus of my treatment would be to provide her with support and adjust her medications.

Prior to our first appointment, I contacted her psychotherapist. We spoke at length. He stated he had established firm boundaries with Barbara. She was not to call him at his office between appointments for any reason. If feeling suicidal or wanting to self-mutilate – a cardinal sign of BPD - she was instead to visit the emergency department. He had given her tools to cope with such impulses and her job was to practice and utilize them! BPD patients are characteristically manipulative. Firm boundaries, like those established by her therapist, are a common method to minimize any manipulative behavior.

At our first appointment, Barbara showed up 20 minutes early. I could hear her pacing in the waiting room. When her appointment time arrived, I called her in. She was tall and slender, even skinny. She was nervous and agitated. Yet well dressed in long sleeves and slacks. She began by saying that she was "at the end of her rope." She felt that no one could help her and said that she felt miserable. I calmed her down a little and asked if she could tell her story from the beginning. She told me nothing I had not seen in her records. Her troubles had begun at around age 14 when she became infatuated with one of her schoolteachers.

He was young and extremely attractive. She began to show her affection, but he kept appropriate boundaries between them. But she saw his action as rejection and found that only by cutting her wrists with a sharp razor could she relieve her anxiety and anger. This non-relationship was followed by several failed relationships including two brief failed marriages.

I now asked about her treatment history and whether any treatment had ever helped her. She said no, adding that "no one understands me". I asked about her progress in psychotherapy with her therapist; she said simply that nothing helped. I reviewed her medication regime with her and suggested some medication adjustments and to continue the plan her psychotherapist had developed which, in my view, was a good one. She left me with the feeling, not unlike the feeling I have about Ms. Bella (Case #1), that I had no way to help her.

Just the next day, as I was leaving my office for the day, she phoned me, sobbing, to say that she was driving on California Street and had just cut her wrist. What should she do? She was probably testing me since I just yesterday had repeated and reaffirmed the rules of her therapist. A trip to ER was in order, and she was close to one. The next morning, I contacted the ER to see if she had shown up. She had not. I instructed my secretary to call Barbara. She answered the phone and told the secretary that she had eventually calmed down. She was OK.

In the coming weeks, I saw Barbara every other week. We worked on adjusting her medications to minimize her impulsivity and her depressed and anxious moods. Repeatedly she called my office during work hours. But the answer was always the same: go to the ER if it was urgent and if not, she was to wait for her next appointment. She was seeing her psychotherapist regularly in addition to seeing me. Her self-cutting behavior continued.

As in many hospitals, ours routinely conducted what is known as "Difficult Case Conferences". In them, a psychiatry resident presents to the rest of the faculty all details of the case assigned to him or her. The ensuing discussion can be quite intense, with new recommendations made. *The conference consensus was that the diagnosis was accurate, suggested one medication change, and to continue with her psychotherapist.* Shortly afterward, I told Barbara that I had discussed her case with other doctors, and she seemed to appreciate the concern. She accepted the recommended medication changes. The case conference concurred with the psychotherapeutic approach in progress.

Two weeks later I saw the patient in what I thought would be another routine visit. But she did not show up for the following visit and could not be contacted. A certified letter sent to her returned informing us that she has moved without leaving a forwarding address.

I knew now that I had been unable to help her.

BPD remains one of the more mysterious and treatment-resistant psychiatric disorders. There exist a few, costly, specialized programs for BPD. *All are in-patient services that routinely begin by stopping all medications and usually last a few weeks.* I had discussed them with Barbara. But she was unwilling to try it. Deep down I suspect she felt none of them could possibly help her. She had suffered too many defeats both in life and in therapy. And she had found no one who trusted her, and in whom she would place her trust.

My Thoughts:

I am a believer in specialization and, more than that, a believer in super-specialization when it comes to matters of assessing and caring for psychiatric disorders. For virtually every psychiatric disorder there exists today a rapidly growing literature on that disorder, one that is helping specialists to *understand* it and work towards a cure. There exist also societies of disorder specialists who regularly attend conferences with fellow specialists, who share their knowledge with their colleagues and who then return to apply their newly gained expertise in their daily interactions with their patients.

Commonalities exist across all disorders – commonalities of mood, anxiety, psychosis, addiction, and personality disorders - it makes sense to me that a clinician should specialize in one of these categories. But this may not be sufficient because many disorders fall within each category and with largely varied symptoms and treatments. As an example, a clinician specializing in personality disorders may want to further specialize in borderline, paranoid, antisocial, obsessive-compulsive, etc.… disorders. This super-specialized clinician would of course be expected to handle the more difficult patients in his/her field. He or she would in addition educate not only his colleagues but his entire community of clinicians. While it is hard to expect this sort of specialization among general practitioners, I would fully expect it in Academic Centers.

A consultation with such a super-specialized clinician would have been significantly reassuring to me that no stone has not been turned in the effort to help Barbara.

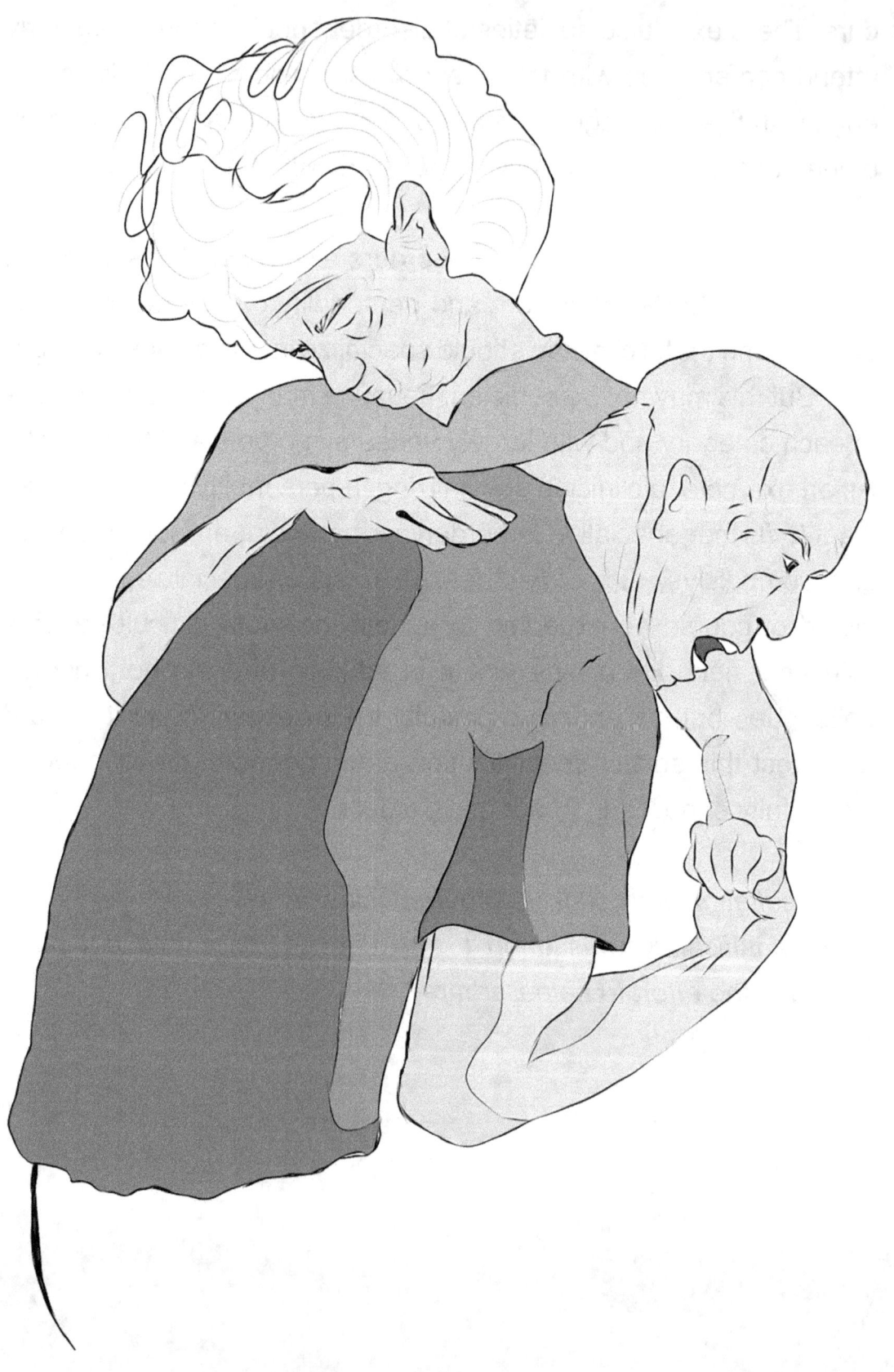

Case Ten

The Unresponsive Schizophrenia Patient Whose Parents Taught Me a Lesson About Trust

In one of my academic positions, I developed and led a specialized clinic for treatment-resistant patients suffering from schizophrenia. One stood out as clearly the most resistant. Mr. Tanner was 32 years old, never married, and never employed. But he had three semesters of a college education. At about age 19 he had begun experiencing auditory and visual hallucinations. Both frightened him. His auditory hallucinations (i.e., voices heard by him but not by others) were usually threatening to him. At times, they urged him to avoid all people because everyone was plotting to kill him.

When I saw him, I noticed in addition that his thought processes were highly disorganized. He had a hard time putting even simple sentences together. In my experience, this was an ominous sign of probable unresponsiveness to treatment. I proceeded to diagnose Mr. Tanner as suffering from Disorganized Schizophrenia. It was no easy diagnosis to make. Because to this day, no treatment has been developed for this variety of schizophrenia.

Following that appointment, I scheduled an appointment with Mr. Tanner for every four weeks. He would come accompanied by one of his parents, though usually frequently by his father.

Mr. Tanner had never harmed anyone. But in one of the visits, my staff and I witnessed how frightening he could be. On this occasion,

Mr. Tanner and his father arrived a few minutes before the appointment time. The nurse called them in. The routine was to check on Mr. Tanner's blood pressure and take his temperature. He declined both. This was not like him. The nurse asked me if we could proceed with the appointment, and I said yes. Father and son entered my office, but Mr. Tanner refused to take a seat and stood next to the door. He looked agitated and frightened as well. I tried to calm him down, asking what was disturbing him. But he didn't respond, just looked at me suspiciously. So, I turned to the father and quietly asked him if he had seen any changes in his son's condition. There were none that he could think of. I then turned to my notes from the last visit and began talking to the father about his son's medications. But just then Mr. Tanner opened the door and stormed out of my office, slamming the door behind him. I ran out of the office with Mr. Tanner's father to find the son standing at the nursing station with the clinic staff, looking frightened and standing at a safe distance from him.

Feeling confident of my relationship with Mr. Tanner, I approached him slowly and said that he could leave if he wasn't feeling well today. In response, he began moving towards the door and as he did, I signaled to the staff that it was OK for him to leave. The father looked at me, apologized, and said he would take his son home and reschedule the appointment. I asked if he felt comfortable taking his son home and he reassured me that he did. So, he left. I instructed the secretary to call the father in an hour to ensure that they had made it home safely.

The rescheduled appointment occurred in eight days. Again Mr. Tanner was accompanied by his dad. He was calmer this time and, once seated in the office, he began in his disjointed way to apologize for his behavior during his last visit. Between his last visit and this one, I reviewed his medication history and come up with a few suggestions to discuss with the father. He and I did so and then agreed on a somewhat different course of action.

Weeks passed and months passed by – 18 months altogether - with no discernible improvements, unfortunately. But the Tanners never missed an appointment. And they always followed my recommendations. But then there was a change, this time on my end. I received and decided to accept a job offer from a prestigious research university. Now I had to inform the Tanner family. The secretary called to tell Mr. Tanner senior that this would be the last time I could see his son.

The whole family came to the final appointment, father, mother, and son. I began with an apology, saying that I would miss seeing them but that I could not pass up an opportunity to do the kind of research I longed to do. It was the father who responded first. He said he was so sorry to see me go but wished me the best of luck. Now the mother began to cry. I could not see why, given that I had never been able materially to help their son. I was puzzled and said so to the father. He looked me in the eyes and stated, "Dr. Boutros, we know for a fact that you had our son's welfare and interest at heart." He continued, "Once when we called your office and were told that you are away from the office attending a scientific conference, we knew that you were looking for the kind of new information that might help our son". He concluded, "My son and both of us as well trust you and appreciate above all your openness and frankness."

This was a major lesson. Trust has been a major component in this therapeutic relationship. I felt honored that I had been able to earn it.

PubMed

Treatment-resistant schizophrenia (TRS) represents a major clinical challenge. The broad definition of TRS requires nonresponse to at least two sequential antipsychotic trials of sufficient dose, duration, and adherence. Several demographics, clinical, and neurologic predictors are associated with TRS.

My Thoughts:

There is no doubt in my mind that our knowledge about what we now call "Schizophrenia" remains extremely limited. Based on my observations, research, and supported by current literature, there may be five or even ten different entities, that we are presently unable to differentiate from each other with confidence.

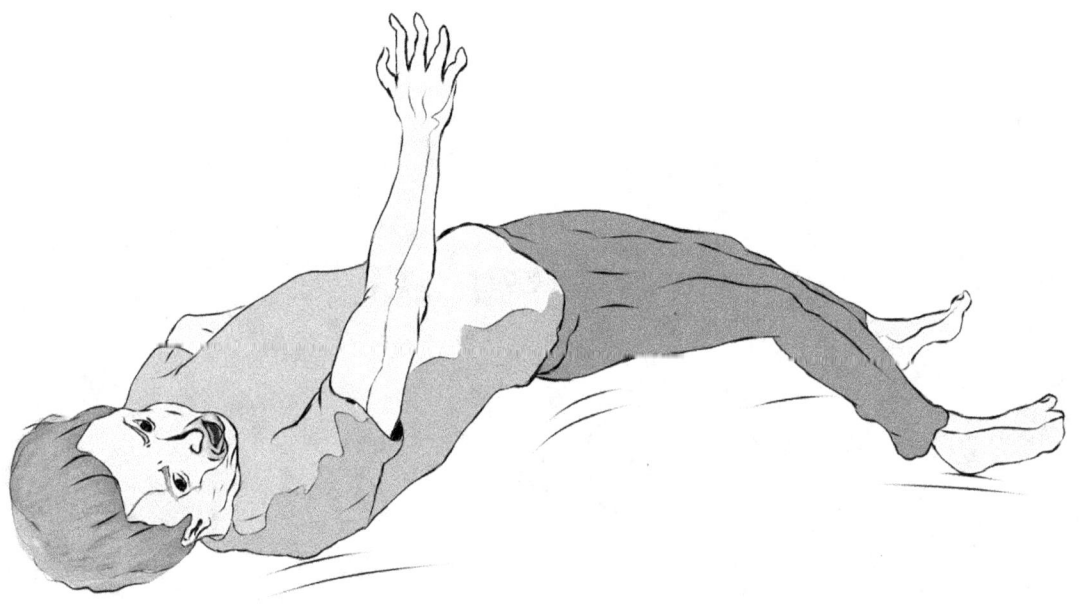

Case Eleven

It's All in Your Head, Sir

As I've already mentioned, I have held joint appointments in the departments of Psychiatry and Neurology at several hospitals. These dual positions made me the frequent recipient of referrals from colleagues in both fields who were puzzled about the nature and hence the treatment of various complex afflictions. Were these afflictions mental and psychological or were they physical and neurological? In certain fairly common cases, this question would arise because the patient's presenting symptoms – debilitating ones like paralysis, numbness, blindness, deafness, or seizures – to all appearances seemed to be physical in origin or stemming from injury or impairment to the nervous system. But in these cases, no clear cause in the patient's life history for these symptoms could be found other than that the patient had been under severe stress from a psychological or physical trauma prior to their onset. Frequently the patient's affliction, upon completion of neurological testing, would turn out to be a psychiatric (not neurological) condition known as a *Functional Neurological Disorder* (FND) or *Conversion Disorder (CD)*. Neurological tests have confirmed the normal health of a patient's neurological system. Having confirmed the absence of a neurological disorder, the neurologist is likely to refer the patient to psychiatric care.

The term "functional" may sound strange, but it conveys the idea – the certainty - that the symptoms of this affliction, however real to the patient or observers, are neither faked nor feigned.

Here is where physicians trained in both psychiatry and neurology are qualified to help FND/CD patients. Neuropsychiatrists are trained to understand both the mental and (seemingly) physical aspects of FND. As a neuropsychiatrist, I had experience working with FND patients who are feeling the full impact of the *physical* symptoms of afflictions such as blindness, stroke, or epileptic seizures.

That said, the field of neuropsychiatry had and still has a long way to go before it will discover and understand the precise (and seemingly unconscious) mechanisms that cause the debilitating symptoms of FND/CD. Theories about their causes abound. But none have gained wide acceptance, and no consistently effective treatment plans have been developed. Conversion Disorders are therefore known as "orphan disorders" in that neither neurologists nor psychiatrists feel comfortable managing them. That's why my Neuropsychiatry clinic received so many FND referrals. But among them, one patient stood out.

Mr. Paul, a single male, age 40, had a high school education but little success holding down a steady job. Often, he was in trouble with the law and had a lengthy prison record. While in court during his latest trial he had had what looked like a full-blown tonic-clonic (grand mal) epileptic seizure. He had fallen to the ground, begun shaking fitfully, frothing at the mouth, and had lost control of his bladder.

These were the classic symptoms of a grand mal epileptic seizure. Difficult to fake, to say the least! So, Mr. Paul was taken to the emergency room and promptly sent to the hospital's neurology unit for a full workup. This included an electroencephalogram (EEG), which proved negative, showing no evidence of epileptic activity. Mr. Paul was then sent to a specialized neurological unit for more extensive testing over several days. Here he was brain-monitored with the hope of capturing a brain wave recording (i.e., EEG) of an actual grand mal seizure. The specialists at the neurology unit knew that the electrical signature of a full-blown seizure would accompany the clinical manifestation of an *actual* epileptic seizure. When seizures occurring during monitoring produce a brain wave recording that shows no evidence of abnormal electrical brain activity, the testing procedure is considered a full-proof diagnostic test for a *psychogenic non-epileptic seizure* (PNES). During his three-day stay in the neurological unit, Mr. Paul did have a grand mal seizure while his brain was monitored. But this test was negative again. He was then transferred to my care.

The first task of a neuropsychiatrist in cases of FND/PNES is to explain to the patient that the episodes are so real to him and are indeed real and not "just in his head." Their families and loved ones must understand this as well. The next step in Mr. Paul's case was to help him connect prior episodes or conditions of stress in his life to these symptoms. Addressing other underlying psychiatric disorders, which could include depression and anxiety is also crucially important. Known as *co-morbid psychiatric disorders*, these conditions must themselves be accurately diagnosed and treated. The task for patients, psychiatrists, and psychotherapists alike is daunting indeed.

On his first visit, I explained to Mr. Paul and the girlfriend he brought with him neuropsychiatry's limited knowledge about PNES episodes. I assured them both that these episodes weren't all in Mr. Paul's head even though the seizure-like episodes captured when his brain activity was being monitored for three days proved that he was not epileptic. During his stay in the neurological unit, Mr. Paul spoke of an anxiety disorder that preceded his first seizure. This, he was told, had to be addressed. His response, on hearing this, was extreme anger. He accused the neurologist who had referred him to my clinic of completely misunderstanding him. Hearing now from me that talking therapy would be the best course of treatment for his seizures, neither Mr. Paul nor his girlfriend was willing to talk further and asked to leave my office, which they promptly did. I looked around. Suddenly the office felt empty. Painfully so.

Ten days later, I took a call from the emergency room of another hospital in town. Mr. Paul had been brought after experiencing a seizure while walking on a busy street. Learning that I had seen him, they contacted me. I said that Mr. Paul had discontinued treatment in the middle of his first visit with me, adding, however, that I would be more than willing to see them again. Hearing this, the physician in the emergency room managed to convince Mr. Paul to give me a second chance. Hats off to him.

During his second visit, again with his girlfriend, I decided to offer Mr. Paul something new. Would he care to participate as a subject in a research study, now in progress, which was focused on his PNES disorder? The study, I told him, showed great promise of making a substantial contribution to our knowledge about how the brain produces the symptoms he was experiencing.

In this research study, I told him, researchers were observing the electrical patterns of the brain using a new neuroimaging technique for monitoring brain activity called *magnetoencephalography* or MEG. The MEG device, I said, is more sophisticated than the standard EEG. I now had his full attention. I said that where the EEG assesses only the *electrical activity* emitted by the brain, the new MEG technology assesses the *magnetic fields* generated by the brain, hence the *magneto* of its ponderous 11-syllable name.

When I added that his participation in the research study would be at no cost to him, Mr. Paul willingly agreed to participate. And indeed, he was a model participant and was paid for his participation. Once concluded, the study's results were explained to him. The study had succeeded. It had confirmed that the brain activity of PNES sufferers does differ, substantially, from the brain activity of non-PNES subjects who are matched in age, gender, and education.

In addition to seeing me, Mr. Paul was also seeing a psychotherapist. In several psychotherapy sessions Mr. Paul, jointly with his psychotherapist devised simple yet creative ways for him to reduce the stress of his life. Mr. Paul incorporated them into his daily routine and in so doing significantly reduced both the frequency of his PNES attacks and his general feelings of anxiety.

DSM 5 - Disorder Class: Somatic Symptom and Related Disorders

   A. One or more somatic symptoms that are distressing or result in significant disruption of daily life.

B. Excessive thoughts, feelings, or behaviors related to the somatic symptoms or associated health concerns as manifested by at least one of the following:

    a. Disproportionate and persistent thoughts about the seriousness of one's symptoms.

    b. Persistently high level of anxiety about health or symptoms.

    c. Excessive time and energy devoted to these symptoms or health concerns.

C. Although any one somatic symptom may not be continuously present, the state of being symptomatic is persistent (typically more than 6 months).

My Thoughts:

Conversion cases remain largely ununderstood and greatly in need of research. No standard diagnostic test for the disorder has been developed. This deficiency causes vast numbers of patients to be saddled with unnecessary diagnostic procedures, some with possible significant harmful complications. On the other hand, there exists a growing number of neuropsychiatry clinics worldwide where such conditions are being addressed more competently.

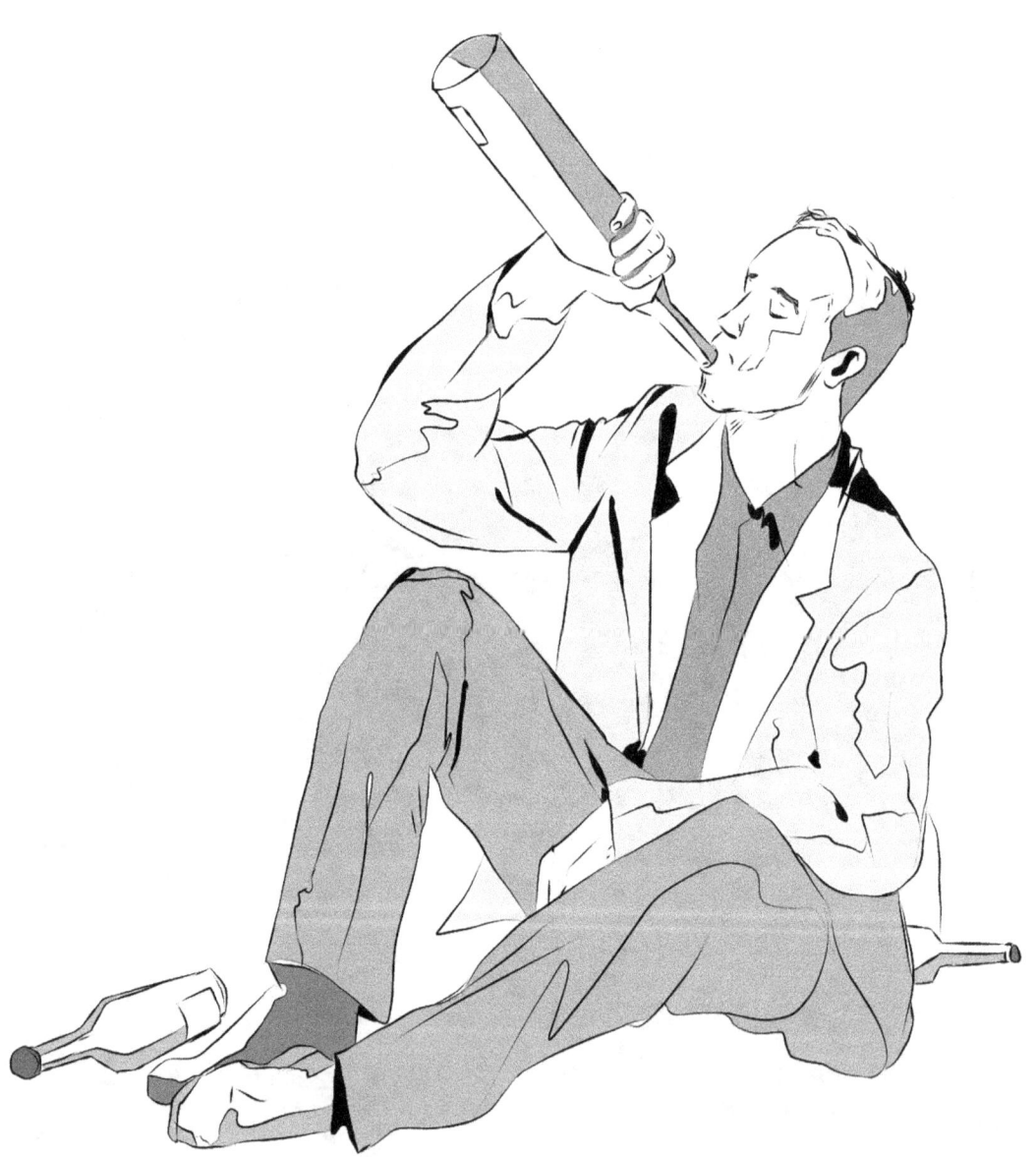

Case Twelve

The Alcoholic in Delirium

Mr. Lance was an alcoholic well known to the emergency room of a major university-affiliated hospital where I was working and teaching in the Department of Psychiatry. He would show up or be brought in intoxicated at least twice weekly, sometimes more often. Indeed, a special alcohol detoxification program had been set up just for him. Mr. Lance had a college degree but was unemployed at this time. He was also a Vietnam War veteran who had seen combat over many months, who had participated in much killing, and had seen many of his buddies killed. He had been diagnosed with post-traumatic stress disorder and was undergoing treatment for it.

But this time, Mr. Lance's visit to the emergency room was alarmingly different. He proved unresponsive to his regular de-tox program. Two hours into his management, his condition was worsening. He was visibly agitated. I was called in. Observing the patient, I decided to bring in the on-duty neurologist. She decided that the patient was in a severe state of alcohol withdrawal (known as *delirium tremens* or DT) and suggested more aggressive management. This called for increased dosages of the standard treatment for his condition found in the class of medications known as benzodiazepines. This class includes Xanax and Valium but now, for Mr. Lance, the medication of choice would be Ativan (generic Lorazepam).

Ativan was administered. But 90 minutes later the patient's condition continued to worsen. His pulse rate was rising, and his blood pressure was fluctuating. I was now seriously concerned. I decided to request a second consultation, this time from my colleagues in internal medicine. The entire group promptly appeared and examined Mr. Lance. Their assessment was that he was in a state known as *iatrogenic delirium* and was being *overmedicated*, not undermedicated. This type of *delirium* is common among adult patients in ICUs and during long hospital stays. Mr. Lance was now in a state of absolute emergency, with death a real possibility. And the question was, from which type of delirium was he suffering? His life hung on the answer (and proper medication) to this question.

Suddenly it hit me that the question would best be answered by means of an analysis of the patient's brain waves via electroencephalography or EEG. From experience, I was familiar with the different brain wave patterns for these two conditions, delirium tremens and iatrogenic delirium. These wave patterns are very different, and I could tell, within minutes of brain wave recording, which one was occurring in Mr. Lance's brain. So, I sprang into action. I ran and grabbed the EEG equipment sitting in my lab and within a few minutes had applied to Mr. Lance's head the sensors needed for the recording. Now I could see his brain waves as they came off the machine in a printout (now the newer equipment display the brain waves simply *on* the screen of the machine). To my amazement, the EEG confirmed not delirium tremens but *iatrogenic delirium.* It disproved the neurological diagnosis and confirmed the internal medicine one. We had been dangerously *over*medicating the patient. Immediately I ordered a gradual lowering of the dosage of Ativan.

With amazement, the staff and I saw the patient visibly improving as his medication tapered off. Within two hours, we felt entirely comfortable removing the restraints that had tied Mr. Lance to his bed. He now sat up and asked for food. Before long Mr. Lance had fully oriented himself to his situation. An hour later, he was transferred to a regular room in the hospital for overnight observation. We all breathed a sigh of relief.

The use of EEG technology in an emergency room in a situation like that of Mr. Lance wasn't just unusual, but, so far as I know, unheard of. The saving of his life required a specialist's knowledge of the different brain waves occurring in these two types of delirium. This emergency room experience changed my life. It made me something of a crusader in the medical community for the more extensive use of relatively inexpensive and completely non-invasive EEG technologies both in and out of the emergency room. As of the time of this writing, I can't tell for sure whether my efforts have succeeded or not. In one important sense they have not succeeded, for I have not seen training in the use of EEG technology included in any of the training programs that physicians go through for the practice of psychiatry.

Alcohol Use Disorder (AUD).

DSM-5: The presence of at least 2 of these symptoms indicates the presence of an Alcohol Use Disorder (AUD).

In the past year, have you:

- Had times when you ended up drinking more, or longer, than you intended?

- More than once wanted to cut down or stop drinking, or tried to, but couldn't?
- Spent a lot of time drinking? Or being sick or getting over other aftereffects?
- Wanted a drink so badly you couldn't think of anything else?
- Found that drinking—or being sick from drinking—often interfered with taking care of your home or family? Or caused job troubles? Or school problems?
- Continued to drink even though it was causing trouble with your family or friends?
- Given up or cut back on activities that were important or interesting to you, or gave you pleasure, in order to drink?
- More than once gotten into situations while or after drinking that increased your chances of getting hurt (such as driving, swimming, using machinery, walking in a dangerous area, or having unsafe sex)?
- Continued to drink even though it was making you feel depressed or anxious or adding to another health problem? Or after having had a memory blackout?
- Had to drink much more than you once did to get the effect you want? Or found that your usual number of drinks had much less effect than before?
- Found that when the effects of alcohol were wearing off, you had withdrawal symptoms, such as trouble sleeping, shakiness, restlessness, nausea, and/or sweating.
- The severity of the AUD is defined as:
- **Mild**: The presence of 2 to 3 symptoms
- **Moderate**: The presence of 4 to 5 symptoms
- **Severe**: The presence of 6 or more symptoms

My Thoughts:

The thrust of the mature years of my academic career has been to develop a subspecialty within psychiatry that is akin to the neurology subspecialty of Clinical Neurophysiology. In the latter subspeciality, a graduating Neurologist who has completed a neurology residency training program is admitted to an advanced training program of one or two years to learn to use electrophysiological techniques including Electroencephalography (EEG), Electromyography and nerve conduction velocity (EMG and NCV) for the diagnosis and assessment of neurological disorders. I am a strong advocate for resident graduates in psychiatry to receive comparable training in these techniques modified to cater to the needs of psychiatric patients. To this end, I have written several books including "Electroencephalography in Clinical Psychiatry" and "Standard Electroencephalography; A roadmap for Neuropsychiatry Research".

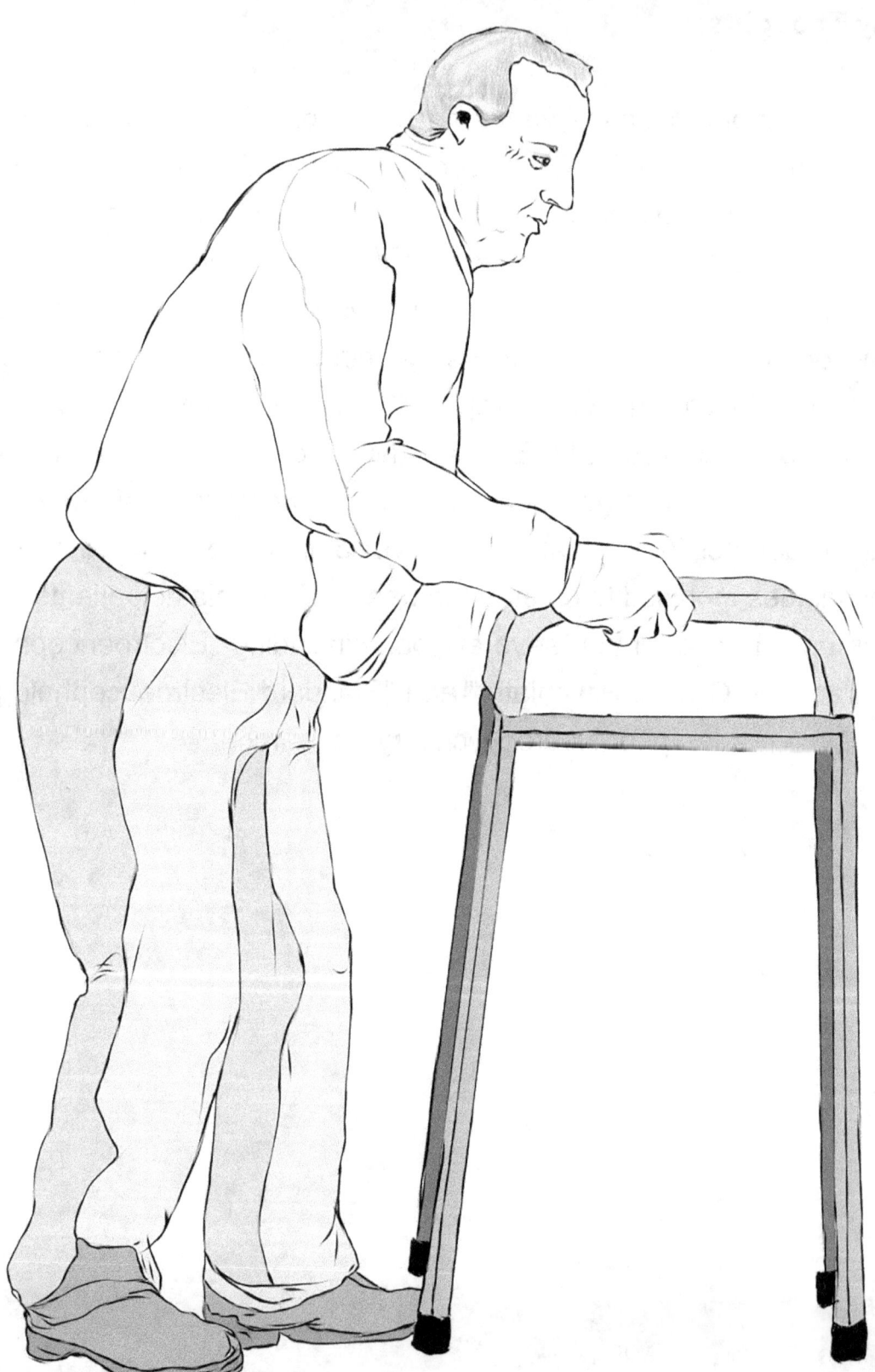

Case Thirteen

Parkinson's or Hysterical Movement Disorder
When Science Simply Could Not Tell

As we saw in Case 11 (The PNES Patient), there exist a number of seemingly neurological disorders for which no kind of testing, whether clinical examination or laboratory testing, can prove or disprove the neurological nature of the disorder. These conditions are then termed *"Conversion Disorders"* in psychiatric terminology and "Functional Disorders" in neurological terminology. The old and off-putting term for conversion disorders was *hysterical conditions*. As we saw in the case of the PNES patient, the mechanism whereby these baffling symptoms develop is unknown to medicine. Treatment is limited to prolonged psychotherapy, not curative but merely adaptive, without any recommended medications.

As also said earlier, my Neuropsychiatry Clinic received numerous Conversion/Functional referrals that fell into the gray area between neurology and psychiatry. But Mr. Zachary was different. A highly educated man, he was also a high achiever and hence a rarity in my experience with conversion patients. Mr. Zachary was well-connected socially and was financially well-off. His marriage was stable, and his children were grown and out of the house. Having traveled widely, he was well-informed and culturally sophisticated, with interests in music and the theater. All this made him a most unusual candidate for a conversion disorder.

Mr. Zachary had been referred to me by a respected neurology colleague who had seen him for several months. I accepted the referral and looked forward to seeing this unusual patient. The notes from my colleague indicated that both the clinical exam and all test results indicated no neurological disorder in Mr. Zachary and, instead, a purely "functional" condition.

On first seeing Mr. Zachary I could not help noticing a constant trembling of the hands and a forward stoop of the gait. Mr. Zachary was using a cane to walk. Speaking with him, I was impressed by the wealth and depth of his knowledge about all kinds of subjects. Thoughtful and measured in his speech, it was hard to think of him as in any way *hysterical. The conversation* soon turned to the reasons for his session with me. I shared my colleagues' preliminary diagnosis of Conversion Disorder. This Mr. Zachary vehemently rejected. I suggested to him that we meet at least twice more to better assess his situation and possibly find a remedy. I promised that I would do everything I could to help him. Hearing this, he seemed relieved. I felt I had managed to earn at least a degree of his trust.

But after four sessions I was still unable to make up my mind whether his condition was neurological (brain disorder) or psychiatric (Conversion Disorder). Speaking with my colleague, I shared my feeling that Mr. Zachary's psychological makeup did not square with the profile of patients with Conversion Disorder. Furthermore, I found no other psychiatric problems in the patient to account for his condition. I asked my colleague to broaden his examination of Mr. Zachary and give me an updated opinion. Given our mutual respect, he accepted my request. The patient was delighted to hear this news and said he was willing to undergo the additional testing required for an in-depth examination.

Two more months passed. Then I received a report from my neurology colleague positively confirming his original diagnosis that Mr. Zachary's condition was not neurological in nature. This news disappointed me, to say the least, and I decided to take another, still broader step. As a member of the Neuropsychiatry community, I worked with nationally recognized colleagues to whom I could turn for expert opinions. I contacted one who taught at a major American university. Mr. Zachary appreciated my doing so and readily agreed to take the trouble and expense of traveling to meet with that expert for further testing and examination.

His appointment with this expert was six weeks away and I told him there was no need for us to meet during that time unless he wished to do so. Six weeks passed, Mr. Zachary traveled out of state to meet with my chosen expert, and ten days later I received the report of the full expert evaluation. And it further confirmed the diagnosis of my local colleague. I was again disappointed, but it seemed that both the patient and the physician had no choice but to accept this assessment and work from it.

For my part, I was willing to do so. After all, it was not hard for me to accept that these two assessments represented the best that science can do at this point in time. But for Mr. Zachary, the task was far more difficult. It entailed his willingness to consider, in extended psychotherapy, that his debilitating symptoms were neither physical nor even neurological in origin. Furthermore, he has to accept that the symptoms were the constructs of a mind that had created them out of a need to avoid the extreme pain of certain prior and deeply suppressed life experiences whose uncovering and healing in therapy could lead to their reduction and possibly elimination. This is the option that I presented to Mr. Zachary. But it was a most challenging option and Mr. Zachary simply declined the offer.

Neither I nor my esteemed colleagues ever heard from Mr. Zachary again.

This case left me wondering if the day will come when a combination of biological tests makes possible *definitive* diagnoses of patients suffering from Conversion Disorders. Currently, as we have just seen here, only neurological tests exist. No biological test existed for me to rule out the possibility that Mr. Zachary's symptoms were biological in nature. Had such a test existed, and Mr. Zachary tested positive on it, it is possible that he would have been open to psychotherapy.

In the PNES case discussed in Chapter 11, the research study mentioned there found a marked difference in the brain wave patterns of patients with PNES and those of the healthy control group. But this study had a small sample. For its findings to qualify for use in a standard diagnostic test for PNES (or any conversion disorder, for that matter), its findings must be successfully replicated by an independent research group in a much larger sample experiment. Once the biological abnormality detected in the small sample study is replicated in the larger sample study, then the findings can serve as the basis of a standard diagnostic test for PNES and

Conversion Disorders. But this road is a long, difficult, and expensive one to travel.

I want to stress here that while conversion disorders cause enormous suffering and expense to patients and their families, they have never been a research priority for the National Institute of Mental Health. This road must be traveled.

My Thoughts:

For some reason, even while accepting the diagnoses of my respected neurological colleagues, a part of me *believed* the patient all along! This case was (and is) an example of an unsettling but unavoidable phenomenon in medicine known as Diagnoses-of-Exclusion. A diagnosis of exclusion means that all other possibilities have been excluded. This leaves the patient with an unsatisfying feeling of receiving a "left-over" diagnosis for which no diagnostic test exists. The answer as I see it is to keep investigating this last-resort diagnosis or condition until we know, positively, what it is and how to definitively diagnose it.

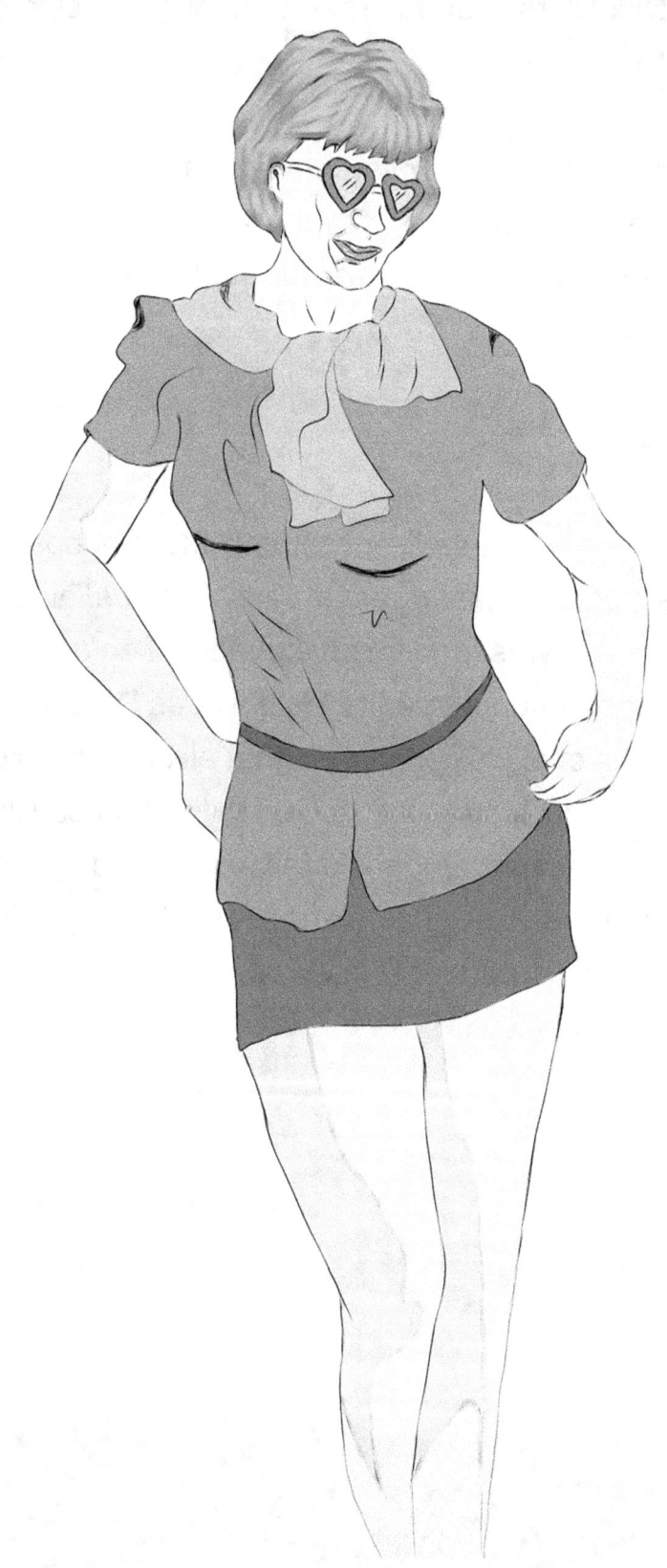

Case Fourteen

The Puzzle of the Sexy Grandma

Ms. Fran, a 74-year-old widow, and mother of two grown daughters, was brought to my Neuropsychiatry clinic by her daughters after they had seen alarming changes in her behavior over the past eighteen months. Previously, Ms. Fran had been a prim, proper, and happy mother of her two daughters and four grandchildren. She had devoted herself to them and had derived much pleasure from being around them, bringing them gifts, and showering them with love.

Over the past 18 months, however, things had changed. It all began with the new bright colors in Ms. Fran's clothes. Then her clothes became more revealing and even provocative. This was quite out of character. Next Ms. Fran began demanding the keys to her car, which she had seen virtually no need to use over the past two years. Puzzled, her daughters complied because their mother's license was current, and her eyesight was fine. Ms. Fran was an active woman and they believed she could drive safely. But then Ms. Fran began going out in the evenings with the car, dressed to kill, and returning late. She wouldn't say where she was going or where she had been.

Alarmed, the daughters followed their mother on one of her outings. Her destination, to their surprise, was a nightclub. They followed her inside and saw her take a seat at the bar, order a drink, and begin flirting with the men around her – younger men. She seemed to be enjoying herself. That evening Ms. Fran ordered three drinks and did not seem inebriated. The two daughters chose not to intervene but simply observed. At around midnight, Ms. Fran left the nightclub and drove safely home.

But once home, Ms. Fran noticed that the car of the daughter who lived with her was missing. Now it was she who was concerned. Her own motherly instincts kicked in as she entered her apartment and found her daughter missing. But now both daughters entered the apartment and, perhaps unwisely, confronted their mother about her behavior at the nightclub. Hearing that her daughters had been following her, Ms. Fran fired back, enraged, that she "was not a child anymore." Precisely the words of an angry teenager. The situation got out of hand, with accusations flying in both directions. Ms. Fran stormed off to her room, locking the door. At a loss as to what to do next, the daughters decided to call it a night.

Two uneventful days went by, with Ms. Fran behaving normally. The daughters relaxed a bit. But on the third night, Ms. Fran once again dressed provocatively and drove off without telling her daughters where she was going. And again, the daughters followed her. This time her destination was a different bar where she struck up a conversation with the bartender. Before long she was in deep conversation with a man in his early sixties. But then Ms. Fran spotted her daughters and angrily demanded that they leave the bar. Seeing no better option, her daughters left. Once home, they stayed up for their mother until 1:30 AM. Then they drove back to the bar.

Ms. Fran had left with the man she had been talking with, as they learned from the bartender, who knew nothing about him. Now frightened for the mother, they returned home. Again, all they could do was wait. And wait they did.

It wasn't until noon the next day morning when Ms. Fran returned home with her clothes wrinkled and her makeup amiss. She

refused to say where she had been. The time had come for professional help.

They called the outpatient clinic at the university hospital where I
worked and described their mother's condition to an intake social
worker who, as it happened, was highly qualified. For two reasons
the social worker decided that I should see the patient. First was the
age of the patient. The second was the fact that the patient had no
prior history of mental health problems. From these two factors, she
knew that this unusual case should be seen by a neuropsychiatrist.

On the appointment day, the daughters showed up with their mother, who had been reluctant to come but was dressed provocatively.
Ms. Fran smiled constantly and responded jokingly to my questions.
She made a point of saying how attractive I was. Her behavior, so
inappropriate in a therapeutic setting, helped to confirm the need
for a full neurological examination. The clinical examination showed
difficulties in what are called frontal lobe signs. Difficulties in this
brain area indicate problems with important functions such as the
ability to learn from mistakes and to plan for the future. It was important now to see an image of her brain, so I ordered an MRI.

Once it was completed, I examined the MRI pictures with the neu-
roradiologist. They clearly showed that parts of Ms. Fran's frontal and temporal lobes were smaller than normal for her age and
smaller also relative to other parts of the brain. I then ordered a third
test known as neuropsychology testing to assess the functionality of
both the frontal and temporal lobes. The results of this test confirmed
to me that Ms. Fran was indeed suffering from a form of dementia
called *frontal temporal dementia* (FTD). Patients with FTD, unlike

patients with Alzheimer's, retain their memory and almost all their cognitive capacities. But they are unable to control their behavior.

In my next visit with Ms. Fran and her daughters, I discussed the report from the neuropsychology testing and the MRI images of the brain, and the accompanying MRI report. Then I had to give them the hard news of my diagnosis. This included the fact that FTD tends to be progressive and no effective treatment for FTD is available. Given Ms. Fran's agitation when any limitation on her behavior is imposed, I prescribed a low dose of a tranquilizer to help her manage it when the need arises. Ms. Fran herself seemed to understand what I was saying, which made sense when one recalled that cognitive functioning was largely intact. Ms. Fran seemed to accept that she would need her daughters' help to keep her safe in the future.

In the following months, I saw her monthly to help her cope with any acute behavioral patterns that arose. A year from the first visit she had to be placed into a full-time dementia care center as her cognitive functioning had deteriorated as well. Despite the inability to halt the progress of the disorder, the daughters appreciated the diligent evaluation and constant support provided by the neuropsychiatry clinic.

PubMed (an internet resource for medical knowledge)

What is Frontotemporal Degeneration (FTD)?

FTD is the most common form of dementia for people under age 60.

It represents a group of brain disorders caused by degeneration of the frontal and/or temporal lobes of the brain. FTD is also frequently referred to as frontotemporal dementia, frontotemporal lobar degeneration (FTLD), or Pick's disease.

How does FTD differ from Alzheimer's disease?

It had different symptoms. FTD brings on a gradual, progressive decline in behavior, language, or movement, with memory usually relatively preserved.

It typically strikes younger. Although the age of onset ranges from 21 to 80, the majority of FTD cases occur between 45 and 64. Therefore, FTD has a substantially greater impact on work, family, and finances than Alzheimer's. (The economic burden of FTD is approximately $120,000 per year, nearly double the amount associated with Alzheimer's.

FTD is less common and still far less known than Alzheimer's. It is frequently misdiagnosed as Alzheimer's, depression, Parkinson's disease, or a psychiatric condition. On average, an accurate diagnosis currently takes 3.6 years.

My Thoughts:

FTD includes several conditions that I could not help with except by offering education and support. During my career, however, I have seen many such conditions become treatable. I am hopeful that effective treatment for FTD will be available before the end of the current decade.

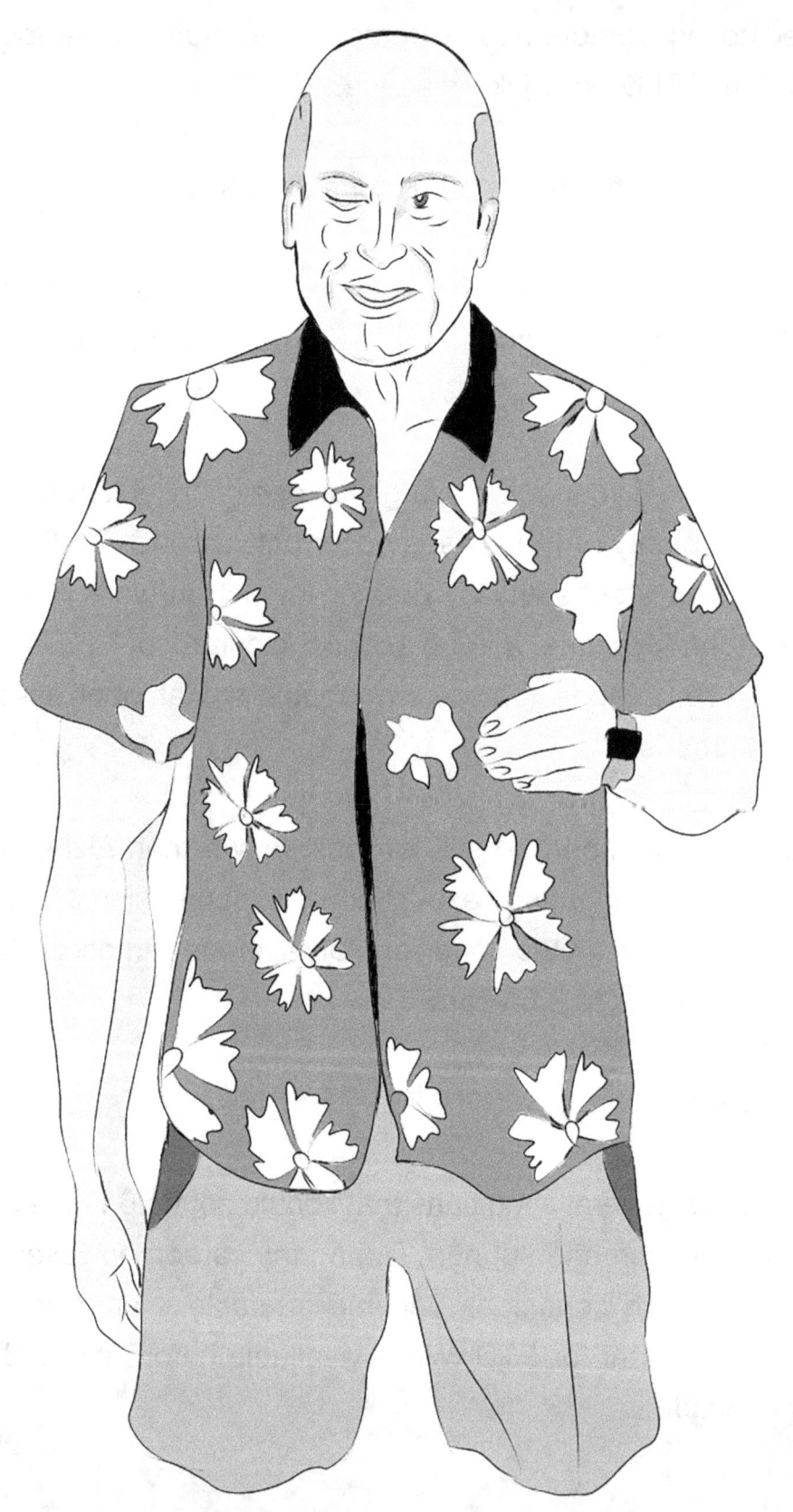

Case Fifteen

The Dirty Old Man

While I was working to help Ms. Fran of Case fourteen with her two daughters, Mr. Floyd showed up at my clinic. His wife and son had made the appointment telling my secretary only that their dad had "gone nuts." Having no medical records for Mr. Floyd, I knew nothing about him. His wife, son, and Mr. Floyd himself arrived on time. But there was a bit of a surprise. Although Ms. Floyd and Mr. Floyd Jr. were dressed appropriately for a doctor's visit, Mr. Floyd appeared wearing a Tee shirt and shorts. In my office, I welcomed them and invited them to be seated.

My large office was furnished with a couch, two comfortable seats, my desk, and an examination bed. This last item was out of place in a regular psychiatrist's office but it served to impress on patients and their families my expertise in Neurology. The walls were covered with certificates earned from residency training programs, fellowships, certificates of excellence in teaching plus my three board certifications in Neurology, Psychiatry, and Clinical Neurophysiology. This last certificate was there to indicate my expertise in performing and interpreting neurophysiological tests such as electroencephalography (EEG).

Both wife and son took seats at the two chairs, but Mr. Floyd, in his early 80s but seemingly in good health, remained standing and looking at me. Angrily, he said, "I don't need to be here, there's nothing wrong with me". In the same voice he continued, though a bit softer, "They want to control my life, or what's left of it, doctor". He then sat on the couch at the farthest point from me. In response, I said reassuringly that I just wanted to get to know him and his family better to see if there was anything I could do to help them smooth out any issues or conflicts.

Soon I learned that some six months ago Mr. Floyd had insisted on leaving home and moving into a senior citizens complex where he had his own one-bedroom apartment. The staff of this housing complex made a point of not interfering with residents' daily lives. They provided breakfast and dinner for residents and arranged group outings and social get-togethers and dances. So far so good, but I still had no idea why this family was in my office.

Finally, the son began explaining the situation. Several months ago, his father had arranged for an escort - a woman - to visit his apartment at the senior complex. Mr. Floyd had paid for her services with a credit card. His wife had seen the bill. A thousand dollars! The son had then inquired at the housing complex and been told by a staff member that his father was becoming more flirtatious and at times acting quite inappropriately with some members of the female staff. He had actually invited a female staff member to give him a massage, he said, "with a happy ending!"

At this point, son and wife had decided it was time for a serious talk. They spent a full day with him including lunch at his favorite restaurant. But once there Mr. Floyd flirted with the waitress and then ordered his food to go, demanding to be driven back to his apartment. Once there, the son went to the bathroom in his father's bedroom.

A stand next to the bathroom stall had a drawer. Curious, the son opened it to see a stack of pornographic magazines.

As in the previous case of Ms. Fran in case # fourteen, I strongly suspected Mr. Floyd's condition to be another case of *frontotemporal dementia* (FTD). There was always the possibility that his behaviors could be manic in nature, which would make them more treatable. But that, in my opinion, was unlikely. While no diagnostic tests exist for manic states, standard tests did exist for FTD, so I ordered three of them for Mr. Floyd: MRI, EEG, and Neuropsychology testing.

I informed the family that these tests would help us understand what was going on and what could be done to help. Mr. Floyd said that he would "humor me" and cooperate with the tests. I indicated my indebtedness for him being so gracious. The family left after I had made all the necessary appointments.

Unfortunately, all three test results came back confirming my worst fears: Mr. Floyd was suffering from progressive FTD. While FTD had not yet encroached on his cognitive functions, it had seriously affected his impulse control capabilities and would continue to do so in the future. I called the family to schedule a follow-up appointment.

They again showed up on time. And this time Mr. Floyd seemed more comfortable in my office. With a big smile, he shook my hands as if we were old friends. "How about it, Doc," he said, "I aced these tests, didn't I?" He stood waiting for an answer. I sat everyone down and explained that the tests unfortunately confirmed atrophy in the frontal and temporal parts of the brain. The condition was known as

FTD and at this time, I had to say, no effective treatment was available. Hearing this, Mr. Floyd angrily declared that I was just another incompetent doctor. "I feel fine, isn't that enough for you?" He then left the room. I apologized to his wife and son about the bad news of the tests. They nodded understandingly and asked what could be done. I explained that Mr. Floyd would need to be housed in the least restrictive environment that would keep him safe. I prescribed a tranquilizing medication to be used sparingly but as needed for agitation.

I then saw Mr. Floyd every other month for two years until the point when his loss of cognitive abilities required that he move to a specialized memory care facility staffed to monitor his behavior around the clock. It was not a happy ending. But the diagnosis, facilitated by neuroscientific testing, was at least accurate and, if nothing else, had spared Mr. Floyd the option of months of unnecessary medications and psychotherapy grounded in an inaccurate diagnosis of manic depression. I am saddened to say that, during my 50-year career, I have seen this error made more than once.

DSM-5

Major neurocognitive disorder, known previously as dementia, is a decline in mental ability severe enough to interfere with the person's independence and daily life. FTD is one of the major forms of Dementia.

This term was introduced when the American Psychiatric Association (APA) released the fifth edition of its *Diagnostic and Statistical Manual of Mental Disorders* (DSM-5).

The updated manual replaces the term "dementia" with *major neurocognitive disorder* and *mild neurocognitive disorder.* FTD is considered a major neurocognitive disorder despite the observation that behavioral control and not cognition (as in memory function) are usually the presenting symptom.

My Thoughts:

The most common error committed by unwary clinicians is diagnosing the condition of Mr. Floyd as a manic state of bipolar disorder. While delaying the correct diagnosis does not affect the course of FTD, the prescribed medications for bipolar disorder have undesirable side effects, particularly for Mr. Floyd's age group. As most psychiatrists are not trained to diagnose or manage dementia, a Neurology consultation is sufficient to prevent this error.

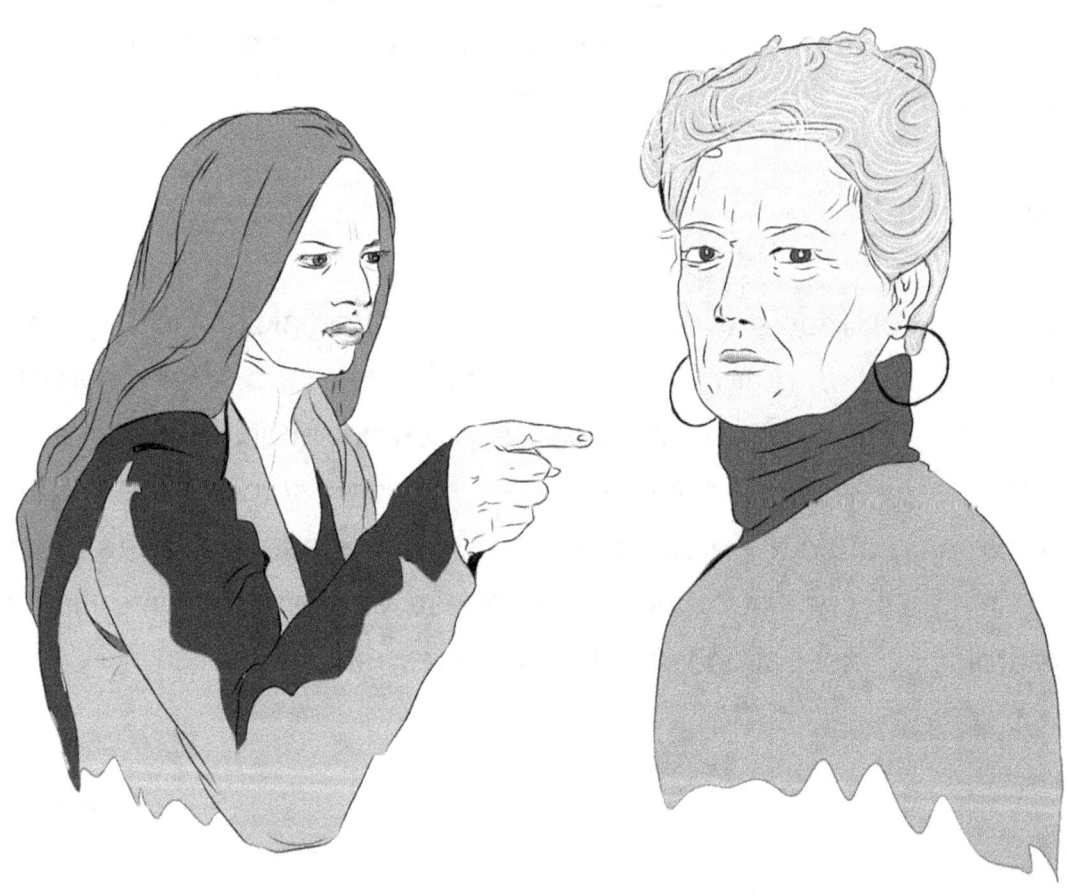

Case Sixteen

The Immigrant Western European Mother and Daughter Who Really Was the Patient?

A call for an urgent appointment came to the secretary of the psychiatry department. The caller stated that her mother was out of control and needed immediate help. It was my turn to take the next referral, so the caller and her mother were scheduled to see me at my very next opening five days away. As a matter of routine, callers are advised to seek help from the emergency room if needed. But on this occasion, the caller accepted the appointment in five days.

On the appointment day, they showed up on time and completed all necessary pre-visit forms, which include several psychiatric questionnaires. The mother, who spoke no English, was helped by her daughter, who spoke English well, to complete the questionnaires. The secretary then brought them into my office. We shook hands and I asked them to have seats. The daughter looked tired. But the mother - the identified patient - looked relaxed and was smiling. Both were well dressed. The daughter started by informing me that her mother, Julia, did not speak English so she would translate for her. This, of course, greatly impeded my assessment. I had no way of knowing how accurately the daughter was hearing me or how accurately she was translating to her mother. I had to rely on her tone of voice, verbal fluency, and body language. I had also to take note of her eye contact with me and between her and her daughter.

But the assessment proceeded. I reviewed the questionnaires completed earlier. These indicated that the mother was in an apparent manic state. But her calmness upon entering my office, her manner of dressing, and her calm voice made me doubt this assessment.

During the assessment, I learned that the daughter, already fluent in English, had accepted a very advantageous job offer and moved to the USA with her mother about four years ago from a western European country. Divorced and with no children, the only obstacle to her relocating to the U.S. was her mother, who lived with her and strongly objected to the move as she did not speak English and would have to leave all her friends behind.

However, the daughter had pressured her mother to move to the US, claiming that Julia would live in the excitement of a big city. Julia, (the mother) suggested, however, that her daughter come to the US alone and leave her in a senior citizen's facility. Such facilities in their country are among the best in the world. In addition to complete privacy, they offer social and educational activities. Country tours and cruises are included. Medical and financial support are also part of the package. But the daughter could not bear the thought of leaving her mother back in the old country alone.

Upon arrival in the US, there was indeed excitement at first. The daughter found an apartment in a high-rise in the center of the city. Things were looking good for the first few months as the daughter settled into her new job routine. And Julia enjoyed exploring on foot the area surrounding the apartment. Some fun stores and a coffee shop were nearby. But no one spoke her language. And soon boredom began to set in even though she was doing her best to keep occupied knowing that she was helping her daughter succeed.

But then everything changed one afternoon when an older lady was mugged in the immediate vicinity. Rushed to the hospital, she did not survive. The daughter now feared for her mom. Yet Julia was not worried in the least. Still, her daughter began limiting her activities. And the limits increased. Julia became resentful. Then things came to a head when the daughter forbade Julia from *ever* leaving the apartment except in her company. With her daughter at work, Julia was now dependent on American TV, which at that time had no channels in her language.

One day the daughter was in a hurry and forgot to lock the door of the apartment. Bored, Julia took the opportunity to get some fresh air. Walking down the block she felt comfortable and was enjoying herself. At her favorite café, she sat down to a cup of coffee and a slice of cake. Then she continued walking, though further from home. Feeling tired, she suddenly realized she didn't know where she was. She couldn't remember her home address or her daughter's phone number. Mortified, she tried finding her way back home, but without luck. She ended up sitting on the curb in front of a large department store.

After work, her daughter returned home. Finding her mother missing, she lost control and began shouting – but no one was there to help her. Having no car, she started walking the streets in desperation, asking people if they had seen her mom walking around and looking lost. No luck. She now had reason to fear the worst.

But after two hours of walking, she had luck. She spotted her mother sitting on the curb, crying. But instead of relief and joy, she was overwhelmed by anger and yelled at her mother all the way home. Once there, Julia demanded that her daughter let her return to her home country and to a senior citizen home there. The daughter would not hear of it. Instead, she took care to lock her mother inside before leaving for work. Julia could not stand captivity. She began looking for ways to escape, even trying to climb out a window. She was now crying during the day, and mother and daughter were barely on speaking terms. It was now that the daughter called my office, having decided that something was wrong with her mother.

This much I was able to elicit from the daughter with her mother's apparent assent. Needing to speak directly and privately with Julia in order to complete the assessment, I now arranged for a meeting with Julia and a professional translator with mental health expertise. Julia and her daughter showed up as before. I asked the daughter to step outside in order to give her mother the freedom to speak. I assured them of the absolute confidentiality of anything her mom would say. Alone with me, Julia confirmed everything I had already gathered. Then the translator informed me that she had seen in Julia no abnormalities of speech, emotion, or cognition. I then asked Julia if she could go into some detail about the senior citizen facilities in her home country. She was glad to oblige. She started by stating that there are no facilities in the US that even come close to the level of sophistication and service of the facilities back home. She had subscribed to a newspaper in her language which printed a detailed report about senior citizen housing in the US. The report was anything but flattering! She spoke for ten minutes and became emotional in expressing her desire to go back to her home country where she could enjoy more freedom, make new friends, and speak her own language again.

I escorted Julia to meet her daughter in the waiting room. I conferred privately with the translator who, like me, had seen no indications of any form of mental illness in Julia. This left us thinking that the problem might be with her overprotective daughter, who herself seemed free of any psychological abnormalities. We called the daughter and shared our recommendation that she let her mother return to her country and stay at the senior citizens' facility of her choice. The daughter would call her twice weekly and visit her at least twice annually. It was a bitter prescription for the daughter, but much to the delight of her mother, she agreed.

My Thoughts:

While I always stress the need for objective, laboratory-based diagnostic tests for psychiatric disorders when called for, no need for such testing arose in this case. Both the expert translator and I saw no evidence of mental disorder in either mother or daughter. Had there been disagreement between us, or had the daughter insisted that something was wrong with the mother, such tests would then have been in order. While useful and widely available, most psychological tests are still language-dependent, which would have presented an obstacle in the present case.

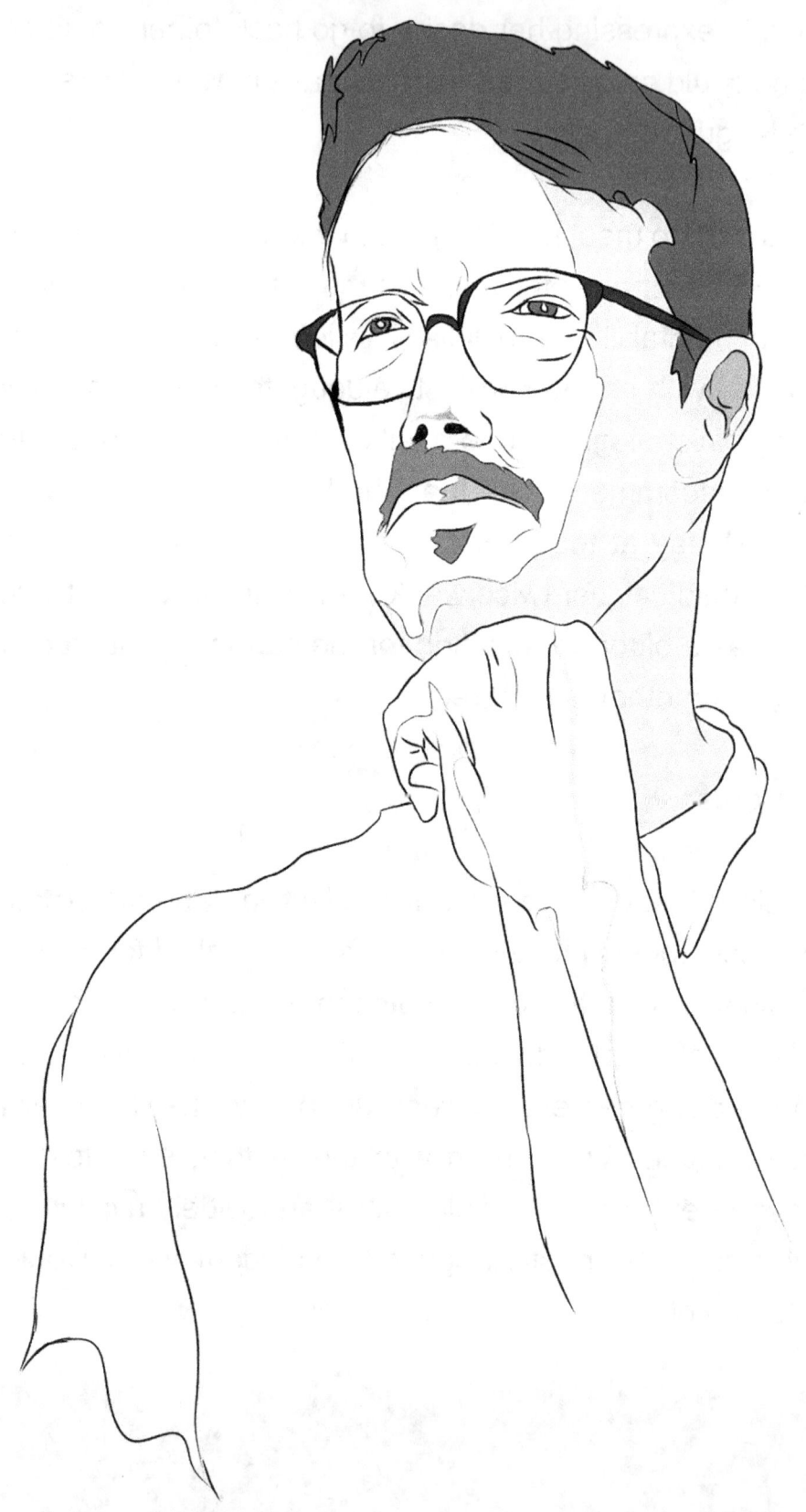

Case Seventeen

The Lawyer and the FBI
Delusional Disorder I

Delusional Disorder (DD) syndrome is a fascinating yet debilitating psychiatric condition. A person suffering from DD remains perfectly sane in all respects except for a single, firmly entrenched, delusional belief. *The delusional belief is not a simple wrong understanding of one fact, but a complex and* systematized *set of beliefs that are completely unsupported by any factual evidence and are not shared by the person's closest acquaintances. The most common of such delusional systems is a conspiracy to harm the individual with many agencies or individuals involved.* The individual can function normally and even succeed in all aspects of life – but only if they can avoid any mention or confrontation with their delusion. Amazingly, they cannot do that, let alone examine their own belief structure, so their delusional belief invariably gets them into trouble, which (with luck) leads them to the office of an understanding psychiatrist. I must preface this case by saying that Delusional Disorder is neither fully researched nor well understood by psychiatrists and treatments available for it even today, as of the writing of this book, are not fully satisfactory.

Mr. Wade was a 44-year-old lawyer employed by a mid-size practice in town. He had been married for five years to his second wife. His first marriage lasted three years and ended because, as he told me, "We grew apart." Mr. Wade was convinced to a certainty that the FBI and other police agencies were after him for reasons utterly unknown to him. He also believed that these threats were responsible for the repeated misfortunes in his life. This, he maintained, was the only plausible explanation for his troubles. He seldom talked about this issue with others but did confide in his current wife. She could not agree with him and instead faulted Mr. Wade. This he flatly rejected. The topic had become a cause of serious friction between husband and wife.

As their arguments got louder and stronger, Ms. Wade insisted that her husband see a psychiatrist. Resentfully, he finally acquiesced. On the appointment date, they both headed to a psychiatrist's office (not mine). As they were about to enter the building, Mr. Wade suddenly insisted that an FBI agent was standing around the corner, possibly to film him entering a psychiatrist's office. So, he refused to enter. Instead, he crossed the street, grabbed a total stranger waiting for a bus, began shaking him, and demanded that he fess up that he was an FBI agent! The frightened stranger pleaded he had no idea about what Mr. Wade was talking about. Mr. Wade had lost all control, he was having a psychotic episode. Loud and threatening, he attracted a nearby police officer who tried to calm the situation. Whereupon Mr. Wade accused the policeman of being "in on the conspiracy," which led to his arrest.

Three weeks later he appeared in court, which mandated that he see a psychiatrist for evaluation, and this led him to me. I knew that the only other disorder that could present symptoms like these was schizophrenia. Mr. Wade, however, clearly did not meet the diagnostic criteria for schizophrenia when we met. So Delusional Disorder struck me as the only possible diagnosis. But when someone shows up with a new behavioral change in my practice, I make sure it is not due to a brain disorder such as trauma, tumor, or epilepsy. But the tests for Mr. Wade all came back negative, which left us with the diagnosis of Delusional Disorder.

Mr. Wade's initial ability to be completely rational as long as we did not touch on his delusion simply amazed me. He exerted every conceivable effort to keep it from coming up but consistently failed. Speaking with his wife, she confirmed this observation. She told me that if her husband "could just see that his fears are unreal, our problems would all disappear." But interestingly, she added that "It seemed as if he was under some kind of internal pressure to bring his fears up with me even when I tried to avoid them". This was useful. It prompted me to try a two-prong approach to helping Mr. Wade. First, I started an antipsychotic medication that is widely prescribed to treat all forms of psychosis. Then I referred Mr. Wade to a trusted colleague for psychotherapy. For my part, I continued meeting with him every other week with a view to trying to help him resist the urge to talk about his delusion, with his wife, especially.

As our sessions progressed, Mr. Wade seemed to be under less pressure to bring up his fears. On our tenth visit together, I hoped to spend the entire 30-minute visit talking about anything but his delusion. This he did! At no time did I detect any trace of any irrationality. I thought, and his wife later concurred, that between the medications and the therapy her husband was doing much better. I continued to see him monthly over the next year with no further significant change in his condition. The delusion, I knew, was still present in him, but he was now able to suppress it. I had to warn Mr.

and Ms. Wade that it could resurface at times of stress. When they relocated to a different state, I no longer heard from them. But I felt their chances for a fulfilling life had significantly improved over the past year.

DSM-5 criteria for Delusional Disorder.

    A.   Non-bizarre delusions (i.e., involving situations that occur in real life, such as being followed, poisoned, infected, loved at a distance, deceived by spouse or lover, or having a disease) of at least 1 month's duration.

    B.   Does not meet criteria for Schizophrenia.

My Thoughts.

(DD) is one of the least researched and widely misunderstood psychiatric illnesses. I am aware of no clinics specializing in managing patients with the disorder. Personally, I confess I have found DD patients difficult to treat. Once I identified the delusional system of the particular patient, my task became to try to help the patient marginalize this delusion and not respond to it. I started by assessing what I termed Delusional Pressure. I defined Delusional Pressure as the degree of the urge under which the patient found him/herself compelled to talk about or behave according to the tenets of the delusion. Usually, upon presentation or referral, the delusional pressure is at a maximum. Regardless of how hard I try to change the topic away from the delusion, the patient, until properly medicated, is unable to leave it.

In my experience, trying to reason with Delusional Disorder patients about their condition has never helped. Only by adding an antipsychotic medication very slowly and gradually, while providing constant reality orientation via competent psychotherapy, have my patients been able to escape the internal world of their disorder. They could then enter with me into the external world from which they may be able to free themselves from their delusion, often to a considerable extent. Having never seen a patient *fully* cured of DD, I consider it a fair success when the patient is able no longer to bring up the delusion with me in conversation – even when I try to get him or her to do so. The few times when I tried to lower a patient's medications, such as when the patient sounded much improved, I found, sadly, that delusional systems promptly returned.

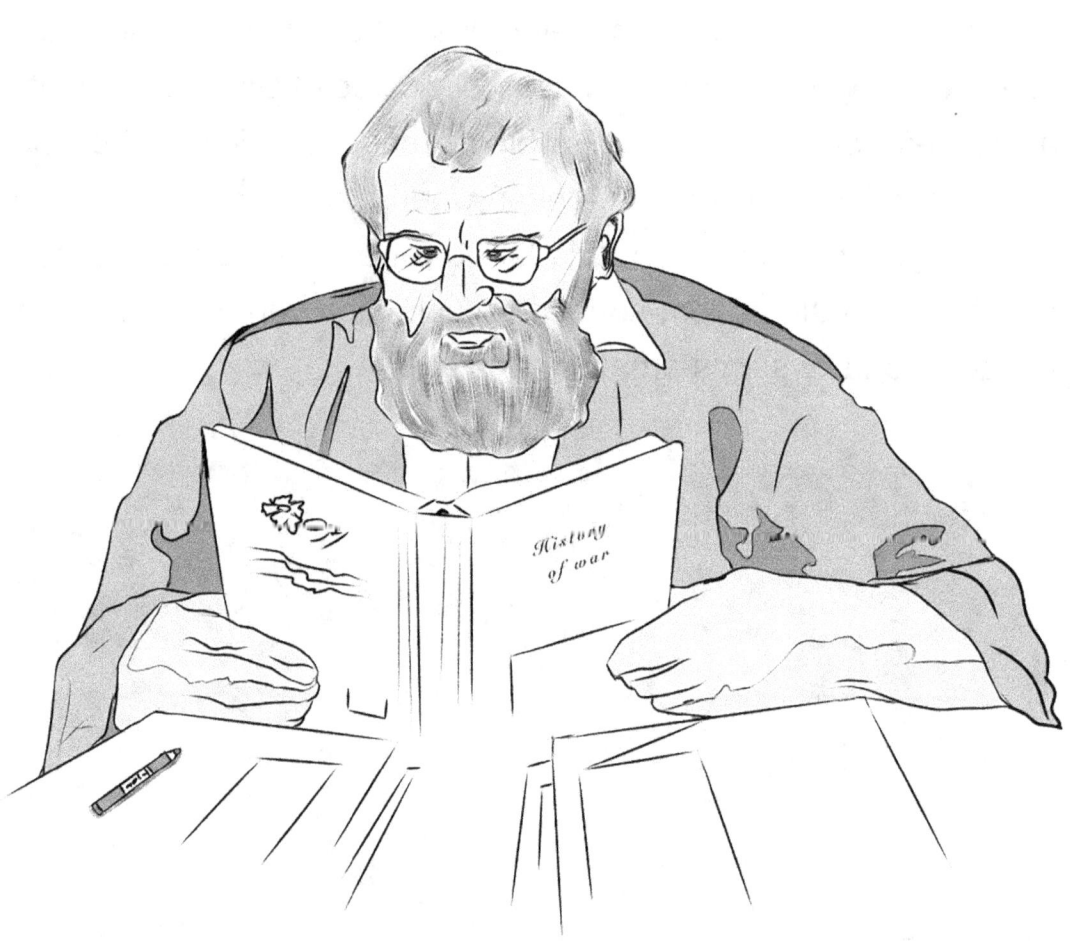

Case Eighteen

A Patient I Could Not Help
Delusional Disorder II

Here is the second case of Delusional Disorder (DD). This time I could not help the patient despite my best efforts. Mr. Xavier was 79 years old when I first saw him. He lived in a long-term facility for chronically mentally ill people who had proved to be unresponsive to all prior treatments.

Knowing the difficulty of treating DD, I still had high hopes after my first interview with Mr. Xavier. His speech was unusually fluent, especially so considering his age. He held an advanced degree in a most challenging field – mathematics - from a major university. He spoke intelligently about his firm (if grandiose) belief that he had discovered a mathematical equation capable of enabling all humans to communicate directly without phones, computers, or other devices. It sounded like a form of telepathy. He had begun developing his formula some five years earlier after retiring from his US government job as a mathematician. In a matter of weeks, he had satisfied himself that his formula for global, device-free communication was correct. So, he wrote a detailed prospectus and sent it out to a number of prospects he hoped would be interested in creating this breakthrough new mode of human communication.

But his efforts met with complete rejection. Mr. Xavier then began to suspect that something was amiss. He first suspected his former employer, the US Government. Sensing a conspiracy, he wrote letters of inquiry to the directors of his former workplace. Responses to his letters - promises to "look into it" – were disappointing and this of course only deepened his fears. Now his letters became threatening. So much so that (long story short) he was eventually arrested and sent to a closed facility for psychiatric care. As with most DD cases, the twofold mainstay of Mr. Xavier's treatment was antipsychotic medications and enrollment in psychotherapy, with the goal of strengthening his ability to adjust his paranoid delusional thinking to a non-threatening reality. Mr. Xavier had resided at this facility for two full years before I met him.

At our first meeting, he began by showing me the prospectus for his formula. It was full of mathematical formulas that I, by no means a mathematician, could not hope to decipher. This gave me no way of knowing whether these complex equations were real mathematics or gibberish or something in between. Yet I took a very close look at them while acknowledging that I was in no position to understand let alone assess them. I felt a bit of relief when Mr. Xavier voiced his sincere appreciation for my interest.

On the next visit, he was brought to my office by the nursing staff. As I mentioned earlier, my office walls were adorned with certificates indicating my training programs, various professional certifications, and memberships in a number of prominent scientific organizations. Before sitting down, he examined each certificate and asked pertinent questions about what each one meant and how difficult it had been to obtain. He was especially impressed by the certificates confirming expertise in research. This, I hoped, might give me enough stature with him to discuss his delusional belief system with credible authority.

As in the previous DD case with Mr. Wade, Mr. Xavier was sane in every aspect of his cognitive and emotional functioning as long as the topic of his delusion was avoided. I decided to spend our second and third sessions developing the trust that might make for a successful therapeutic relationship. During these sessions, I affirmed my confidence in his intelligence and thoughtfulness with the hope that he, in return, would place some confidence and trust in me and in the therapeutic process. I enjoyed these two sessions with Mr. Xavier and made a point of telling him so.

At our fourth session, however, I changed tactics. I asked him how he saw the fact that he was living at a psychiatric facility with little freedom. To my dismay, this got him talking about his delusional beliefs and nothing else. I was powerless to change the topic. So, I just listened. Time passed and so the fourth session was over. Yet Mr. Xavier again indicated his appreciation of my willingness to hear him out.

During my ensuing weekly sessions with Mr. Xavier, I tried to get him to accept that the world – the prospects he has contacted about his formula – was not equipped to see in his formula the merits he saw in it. He appeared to grasp this point without feeling threatened. I had an inkling of hope. I saw to it that he was being properly medicated.

My plan now was to help him accept that his discovery was not attracting interest from funders because it lacked scientific verification. And if this plan didn't succeed, my backup plan was to help Mr. Xavier acknowledge that his ideas might simply be too ambitious for others to grasp them, and, if so, he no longer needed to press the world to accept them. He could keep them safely to himself, as had many great thinkers before him, perhaps leaving it in a format that was accessible to future mathematicians. But alas, even that was too much to ask.

A year passed by, and Mr. Xavier had not improved in any measurable way. I continued modifying his medications hoping for a miracle, making changes by professional intuition, not by science, since DD research is so sparse. I was now leaving the city to accept a new position in a different state. Regretfully, I left Mr. Xavier with the same symptoms as when I had first seen him. He was saddened to see me go, for if nothing else we had shared the pleasures of companionship. I write about him now out of disappointment with the lack of scientific research that could have enabled psychopharmacology and/or psychotherapy to help him much more than it had.

WIKIPEDIA: The prevalence of this condition stands at about 24 to 30 cases per 100,000 people while 0.7 to 3.0 new cases per 100,000 people are reported every year. Delusional Disorder accounts for 1–2% of admissions to inpatient mental health facilities. The incidence of first admissions for Delusional Disorder is lower, from 0.001 to 0.003%.

My Thoughts:

As of 2022, DD syndrome is far from being understood. Its neurobiological bases have yet to be articulated. Nonetheless, I am confident that science will one day understand DD and be able to treat it effectively. Once we have an idea as to how DD develops in the human psyche, treating it will be a matter of time. Yet, as I said in the previous case, I am unaware of any "advocacy organizations" for those suffering from DD even though some 100,000 Americans suffer from it. Relative to other diseases, however, DD is not that prevalent, which helps account for why public awareness of it is almost nonexistent.

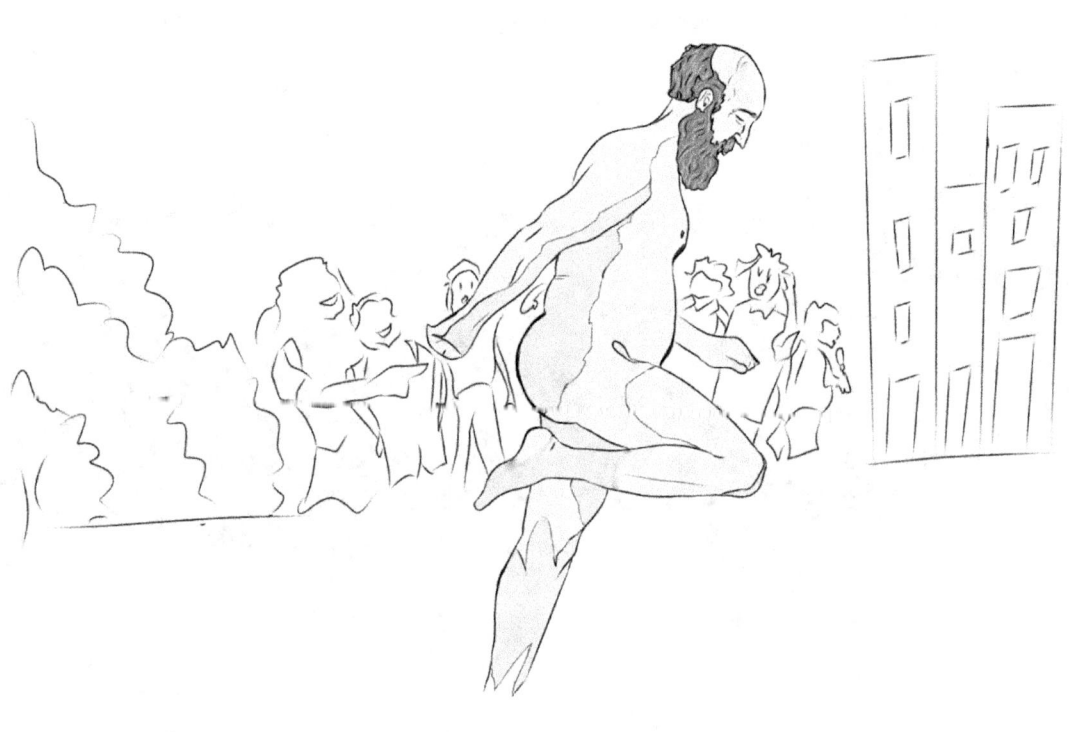

Case Nineteen
The Nude Lude Dude

This case troubled me a great deal, and not because of any difficulty diagnosing it or managing the patient. The cause of my unease came from a third source, closer to home. Mr. Nigel was 52 years of age, divorced, and the father of two. He was unemployed but did have enough income to live independently. The reason for his being committed to a longer-term psychiatric facility was that he had repeatedly run out into the street from his residence with no clothes on while children were playing in the street. During one of these episodes, police were called, and he was brought to a hospital. While I did not work at this hospital, the hospital administration, based on strong recommendation from his treating physician, thought a second opinion from me could be helpful. I agreed, and Mr. Nigel was brought to my office at the University for our meetings.

Upon evaluation, evidence was found for cognitive dysfunction. The origin or cause of his cognitive deficit was then unknown but was thought to be secondary to, or resulting from extensive drug use. While Mr. Nigel admitted to drug use, he could or would not say how extensive his use was. Whereupon the court sent him to receive treatment at the facility where he resided at the time. Apart from a combination of antipsychotic and antimanic medications, no further treatment was given.

Mr. Nigel had been in the hospital for seven months when I first saw him. During these months his condition had gone without a formal diagnosis let alone a treatment plan based on solid clinical grounds. Mr. Nigel was a man of few words. He answered questions in a seemingly straight forward albeit brief, manner. Despite having good eye contact and an occasional smile, I could not develop warm feelings for him! My initial evaluation left me with two observations. First was that Mr. Nigel had repeatedly run naked in the street near his house. The second was that his cognitive impairment was advanced. Knowing that extensive drug use can lead to cognitive deficits, I needed now to find evidence of the extensiveness of drug use in Mr. Nigel. I contacted members of his family. Although they agreed that Mr. Nigel had used drugs, none of them had seen extensive use.

I asked Mr. Nigel about these episodes. They seemed to puzzle him. He said that he liked walking around his apartment with no clothes on. But then an irresistible urge would hit him – an urge to run - and the only place to run was outside. I wondered if epilepsy could be triggering his public nudity. I ran an EEG on Mr. Nigel and sure enough, it detected an epileptic discharge (EEG activity indicative of epilepsy) in his frontal lobe region. This made it likely that his episodes were triggered by this region of the brain

The next diagnostic step would be to refer Mr. Nigel to an epilepsy monitoring unit where his brain waves and behavior would be monitored around the clock. The facilities capable of this simultaneous EEG/Behavior monitoring are both very expensive and exist in tertiary epilepsy treatment centers. In fact, there was only one such facility in town. Two big problems arose. One was the high cost, with the hospital having to foot the bill. Mr. Nigel had no insurance coverage. The second, and more formidable still, was the low frequency of his episodes. In order for this EEG/Behavior monitoring test to be conclusive, an actual episode of the behavior in question had to be recorded both on camera and the EEG within the brief (3-5 days) stays allowed by the hospital for such costly procedures.

To my dismay, the hospital's administration informed me and his physician that Mr. Nigel was receiving adequate treatment at his current facility, adding for good measure that they saw no need for further assessment or additional treatment. I had hoped for better than this for poor Mr. Nigel. Obviously, he had fallen between the cracks of the healthcare system, and my hospital was only widening the gap. Unfortunately, with that, this story comes to an end.

Well, maybe not quite. Let me say first that only a tiny number of epileptics harm others. That said, epilepsy in courts of law has on occasion been held responsible for causing violent acts, including murders. The issue is a contentious one, medical and legal. The legal standard that a violent act is deemed secondary (and to a degree *caused by*) epilepsy is extremely high. The accused must be monitored in a clinical EEG/Video setting for as long as needed in order to capture a full epileptic episode. If captured on video, the episode itself must replicate the actual level of violence for which the accused is being tried. The video must also be accompanied by EEG activity indicating an epileptic seizure lasting throughout the episode. This high standard is seldom met.

My Thoughts:

An epileptic seizure results from overactivity of a certain brain area caused by the failure of the mechanisms that are built-in to prevent such overactivity. When this overactivity originates from the motor region of the brain, the result is simply the familiar process of the patient falling into convulsions. But when the overactivity emanates from other brain regions, such as the frontal lobes, that are concerned mainly with social and cognitive functions, the result can be very bizarre manifestations, such as Mr. Nigel's public nudity. All too often, patients afflicted by these latter manifestations are not properly diagnosed and are relegated to mental institutions.

The tragedy of their situations, and perhaps that of Mr. Nigel, is that when properly diagnosed, effective treatment for this bizarre form of epilepsy is readily available.

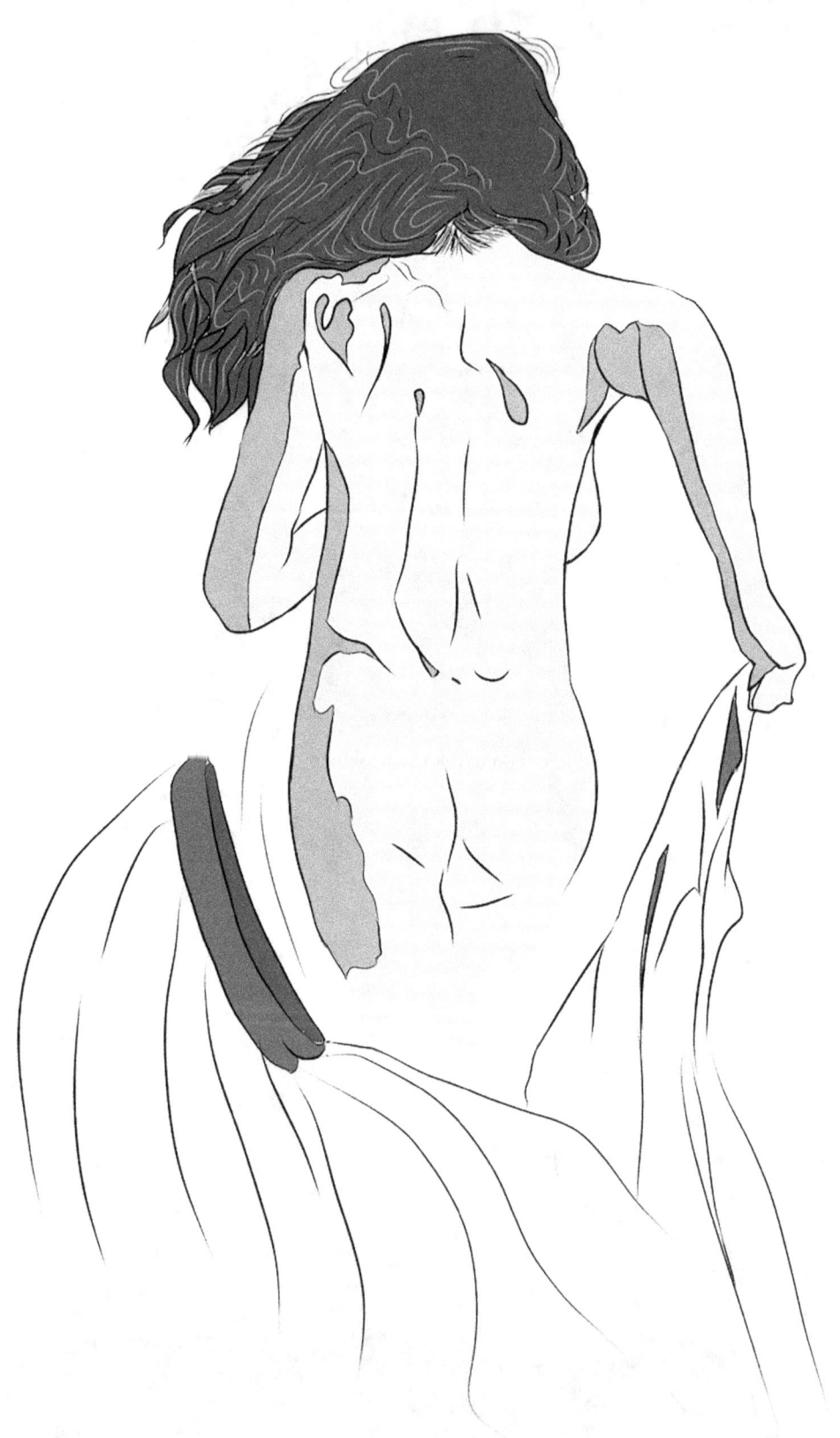

Case Twenty

The Lady Stripper

Ms. Swansen was a 54-year-old single woman who had been homeless for several years. She was admitted to my hospital when I was on duty, so I got to meet her just after her admission. Her history indicated that she had been hospitalized in psychiatric facilities in several states. She was also diagnosed with several psychiatric illnesses some of which were mutually exclusive, meaning (according to the DSM-5 diagnostic system) that they cannot occur simultaneously in the same person because one diagnosis overrides the other.

Ms. Swansen had been variously diagnosed as suffering from Schizophrenia, Bipolar-Disorder, Borderline-Personality Disorder, Antisocial Personality Disorder, drug dependency, and schizoaffective disorder. This brought to my mind the cynical joke about psychiatrists that when a patient sees ten psychiatrists, she will receive ten different diagnoses. This joke probably arose prior to the rise of the DSM system of diagnosing psychiatric disorders, but even with the latest version "DSM-5", diagnosis in Psychiatry remains subjective. As of this writing, psychiatry lacks objective laboratory-based diagnostic tests that facilitate accurate diagnoses in all other branches of medicine.

The immediate reason for Ms. Swansen's current hospital admission was that she (not unlike Mr. Nigel) had completely undressed at a subway station. Her records confirmed multiple instances of this behavior. Brought to the emergency room of a University Hospital, she was promptly placed in a psychiatric facility. Surprisingly, she welcomed this placement despite knowing that it would likely be several months, if not longer, before she will be allowed to leave.

In my initial interview with Ms. Swansen, my challenge was to identify, if possible, the illness she was most likely suffering from. This important first step would of course guide her long-term treatment. Her short-term treatment would address only her current symptoms (i.e., symptomatic treatment). Our first meeting lasted 90 minutes, much longer than my usual diagnostic interviews reflecting the difficulty I faced trying to narrow down the diagnostic possibilities for Ms. Swansen.

In response to my questions, Ms. Swansn confirmed her experience of a wide variety of symptoms suggesting that she was suffering from many disorders at the same time. Oddly, however, **she** did not come through to me as all that sick! In fact, I found the interview quite enjoyable. She was a well-read and knowledgeable person. Her eye contact was fine, and we developed rapport without difficulty. This patient would obviously be a challenge!

Not having detected obvious cognitive deficits during this lengthy initial interview, I saw no need for neurological investigations. Instead, I ordered what is called Psychology Testing. This is a lengthy and standardized interview. There are several standard versions of it, but they all address the possibility of mood, anxiety, psychotic systems, and personality structure. Built into the testing process, significantly, are components that cleverly confirm the truthfulness of patient responses to the questions asked. The results would not come back for a week. During this time, I met with her in two 60-minute sessions with little progress made toward narrowing down the diagnostic possibilities. One thing I had decided was that Ms. Swanson was not suffering from Schizophrenia.

In our second interview, prior to receiving the test results, she told me that she had learned from one of the unit staff that I was born and raised in Egypt. This brought her to the session with a long list of questions about Egypt and its history. Her questions all indicated a high level of curiosity and a genuine desire to learn. She also asked if I could recommend books about Egypt. How unusual, to say the least, for someone with multiple possible psychiatric ailments!

In a few days, the results of the Psychology Testing came in. They were full of all kinds of inconsistencies except for one area; a tendency to greatly exaggerate her symptoms. These results squared with my impressions of Ms. Swansen. And they gave me some new questions to ask her. In our next interview, I tried to zero in on the possibility of a personality disorder that might explain both her exaggerations and her track record of multiple diagnoses. To obtain the focus it would entail obtaining from her a fairly full picture of her life from childhood onward.

Happily, we had already developed a good rapport. She had difficulty talking about her early life even though her story was a sad one beginning with being raped repeatedly - as a child. She had subsequently been placed in foster homes where she was also abused. Of course, I could not verify her account. Later, she said, she was housed in a group home where she felt relatively safe. She liked it there. She did well and her helpful social worker, feeling that Ms. Swanson no longer needed to be in such a controlled environment, began looking for possible employment and an independent living arrangement for her. But it was then that Ms. Swanson first took off her clothes in public . . . for no apparent reason. This behavior of course sabotaged all efforts to return her to normal, unconfined life. It landed her back in a hospital. And this pattern repeated itself. Every time Ms. Swanson felt close to independent living where she would need to protect and support herself, one of her stripping episodes would return her to the safety of hospital confinement.

During one interview with Ms. Swansen she said she had once lived independently for a brief time and had held a job as a waitress. But she never felt safe on her own. Furthermore, she claimed that she had once been raped on her way home from work. When living homeless on the streets she was repeatedly raped and mugged. I felt there was truth in at least some of what she was saying. Clearly, Ms. Swansen found hospitals or even group homes safer than the world outside.

My next meeting with Ms. Swansen was very telling. I informed her of my thought process about her situation. I told her that I did not think she suffered from any diagnosable psychiatric disorder, adding that I felt she had gradually become dependent on the various institutions for safe living. And sure enough, later that day, she had an episode of running naked in the corridor in the unit where she was residing, I surmised that she has misinterpreted my statements to her as a prelude to my discharging her from the hospital.

I met with a social worker and discussed my discoveries with her. I asked if we could arrange for a long-term placement that would allow Ms. Swanson more freedom without the threat of being discharged before she herself felt fully prepared to leave. Ms. Swanson would need much care: a multi-prong approach including work rehabilitation, psychosocial rehabilitation, and close psychiatric monitoring. It was crucial that Ms. Swanson know in advance that she would not be forced out on her own until she requested it.

She obviously did not trust the hospital system. She felt the hospital needed her bed! She had several other stripping episodes before we (myself, the social worker, and her closest nursing staff) managed to convince her that she would be safe with the planned discharge and placement in a new group home. She eventually acquiesced. At the last follow-up, she was doing well in her new home and progressing in work-rehab and psychosocial therapy. And she was succeeding without psychiatric medications.

My Thoughts:

People have feigned illnesses of all sorts for personal gain throughout history. We should differentiate between them and people who suffer from conversion disorders: people, this is, who have no control over their symptoms and who stand to gain nothing whatsoever from their illusory illnesses other than relief from conditions that are causing them extreme psychological pain.

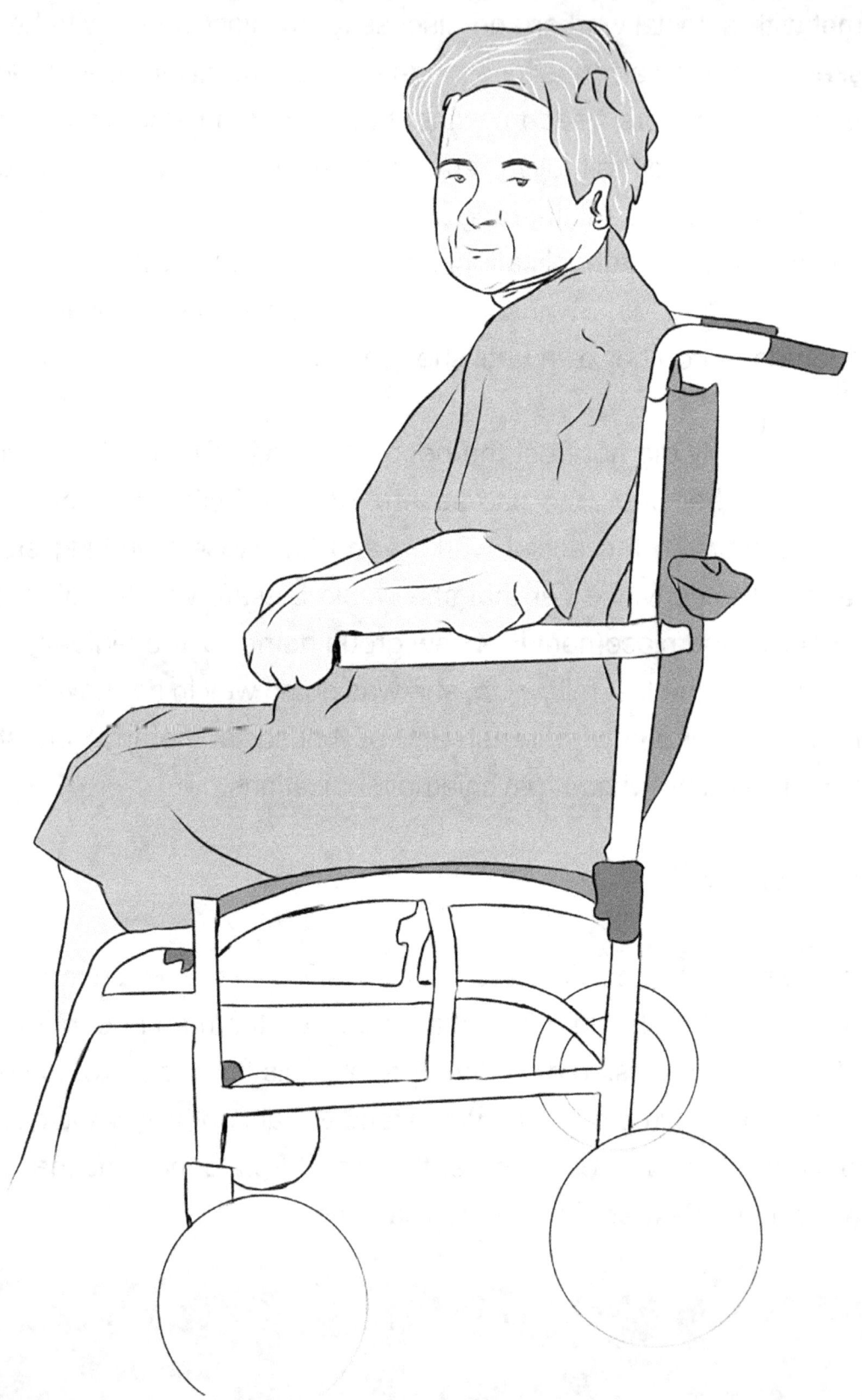

Case Twenty-One

The Demented Woman Who Was
NOT Demented!

In one of my many academic posts, I developed and ran a Neuro-psychiatry Unit. This unit was designed to evaluate and manage patients with manifest or suspected brain pathology (Neurological disorders) resulting in psychiatric manifestations.

Ms. Daniels was a 60-year-old woman, a widow, and the mother of one son. She had been diagnosed with Alzheimer's Disease four years earlier and was now living in a nursing home for the memory impaired. According to the notes from the nursing home, her memory problem had slowly and gradually been worsening. She could still recognize her son but could no longer recognize her home care workers. She had been wheelchair-bound for the past two years.

One morning Ms. Daniels refused to eat breakfast. Then, lunch. The staff of the nursing home became concerned. They tried adding her favorite food, ice cream, to her dinner as an inducement to eat. But she refused to eat anything and at dinner, she refused water as well. So, the staff brought her to the university's psychiatric hospital. Upon her arrival and given her diagnosis of dementia (a neurological disorder), the triage staff wanted to admit her to my Neuropsychiatry Unit. But the Unit's nursing staff, unhappy with this decision, insisted that there was next to nothing that could be done for an advanced case of Alzheimer's like this one. The nursing staff suggested that the triage unit insert a feeding tube through her nose to administer nourishment and send her back to the nursing home. Hospital administration rejected the suggestion and Ms. Daniels was admitted to my unit. Furthermore, Ms. Daniels was what is called a "total-nursing-care" patient. She needed help getting from bed to her wheelchair and going to the bathroom which further increased the unhappiness of the nursing staff.

Rule number one, in managing dementia of any kind at my Unit, was to conduct a full workup in order to be certain that there was no reversible cause for a problem of a deteriorating memory. In fact, there exist a number of neurological and metabolic changes that can result in memory decline and our task was to make sure none of these, if present, were making the patient's condition worse. I instructed the resident physician at my unit to review the patient's history to see if any such workup had been done on Ms. Daniels. If a workup had been done, we would have had to return the patient to the nursing home after her feeding through the nose had been completed.

It took the resident 24 hours to find out that no workup had ever been performed on Ms. Daniels. Her diagnosis of Alzheimer's Disease was based on clinical grounds alone, with no neurological testing. It now fell on my Unit to do the work up. But my nursing staff, still convinced that Ms. Daniels was an Alzheimer's patient, was now doubly unhappy and on the verge of protesting to hospital administration. But we conducted all the necessary tests, and all of them were within normal ranges for the patient's age except for two. The computer-assisted tomography or CAT scan showed mild brain atrophy. The radiologist interpreting the result hedged his interpretation and decided that the test result could possibly agree with the clinical diagnosis of Alzheimer's. The other test was the EEG.

The next morning, after recording Ms. Daniels' brain waves, the EEG technologist came to my office and stated flatly that there was no way this patient could be suffering from an advanced dementing condition like Alzheimer's. The operative word here was "advanced," because it is well-known that in mild cases of Alzheimer's Disease, an EEG test can still fall within the normal range. Hearing this, both of us walked back to the EEG lab anxious to see the test results. On the way, the technologist stated that he would have sworn that this was an 18-year-old person if he did not know better. I was wondering in my head. At the lab, I grabbed the test printout and saw, to my utter amazement, that the record looked exactly as the technologist described. The record was absolutely normal with no hint of any deviations. Ms. Daniels was not suffering from advanced Alzheimer's Disease.

I sat back and asked myself what could possibly be afflicting this patient. The major disorder that is common to be differentiated from Alzheimer's Disease is Major Depressive Disorder (MDD). The EEG of patients with MDD remains normal no matter how severe the depression is. If Ms. Daniels was suffering from MDD, this was good news because her condition was treatable and reversible. The only way to see if this was the case was to treat her for MDD. The nursing staff objected to this treatment and now complained to the hospital administration, demanding an investigation of my conduct. Hearing this, I needed stronger evidence for MDD than just a normal EEG. Here I should add that clinical psychiatrists do not highly value the findings of EEG tests despite significant research showing their diagnostic usefulness.

So, I now turned to a test that is rarely used and is considered controversial: the Dexamethasone Suppression Test (DST). Studies have found patients with severe depression often test abnormally on this test. With it, a small dose of a drug called Dexamethasone is administered. This should suppress the secretion of cortisone in the patient for the next 24 hours. The Cortisone blood level is checked the next morning and again at 4 PM. If both results are low, severe depression can be deemed unlikely. But if one or both levels are elevated, then the patient is considered to be a non-suppressor, and this result favors (though not conclusively) a diagnosis of Major Depression.

Ms. Daniels tested as a highly non-suppressor for *both* blood samples. This result gave me the ammunition I needed to go ahead with treatment for the MDD that I now believed was at the root of her problem. An antidepressant medication was started. My nursing staff was *still* unhappy, but the hospital administration accepted the rationale for what they were now instructed to do. A week passed with no discernable change in Ms. Daniels. The stress was now palpable throughout the Unit; I certainly felt it myself, for I sensed that the outcome of this case would be a turning point for the Unit, one way or the other. On the tenth day, Ms. Daniels said two words to one of the nurses while they were moving her from her bed to her wheelchair. They were "Thank You." The nurse could not believe it. She came running to me with a huge smile to tell me the news. Yet the time to celebrate was still far off if ever we could.

At the beginning of the third week, Ms. Daniels started eating and talking more often. But she was in a psychotic state, seeing body parts all around her and blood on the floor. She was terrified. We immediately put her on antipsychotic medication. Five days later, she was out of her wheelchair and eating on her own. After another week her psychotic symptoms had abated. She smiled and talked to both staff and patients. We discharged her to her son's care. The nursing staff was ecstatic.

My Thoughts:

Pseudo-depression and Pseudo-dementia are especially interesting syndromes as patients of both afflictions present with one disorder when, in fact, they have another. In Pseudo-depression the patient usually suffers from a neurological disorder that causes them to look and act as if they are depressed when they do not feel depressed or even sad. Treatment with depression medications is of no help. Treating the underlying condition, if possible, is the way to go.

On the other hand, in Pseudo-dementia, as exemplified by Ms. Daniels, the patient appears demented when in fact they are suffering from Major Depression. In this case, antidepressants help enormously although the patient may need electroconvulsive therapy (ECT) due to the severity of the depression. Happily, Ms. Daniels did not need ECT.

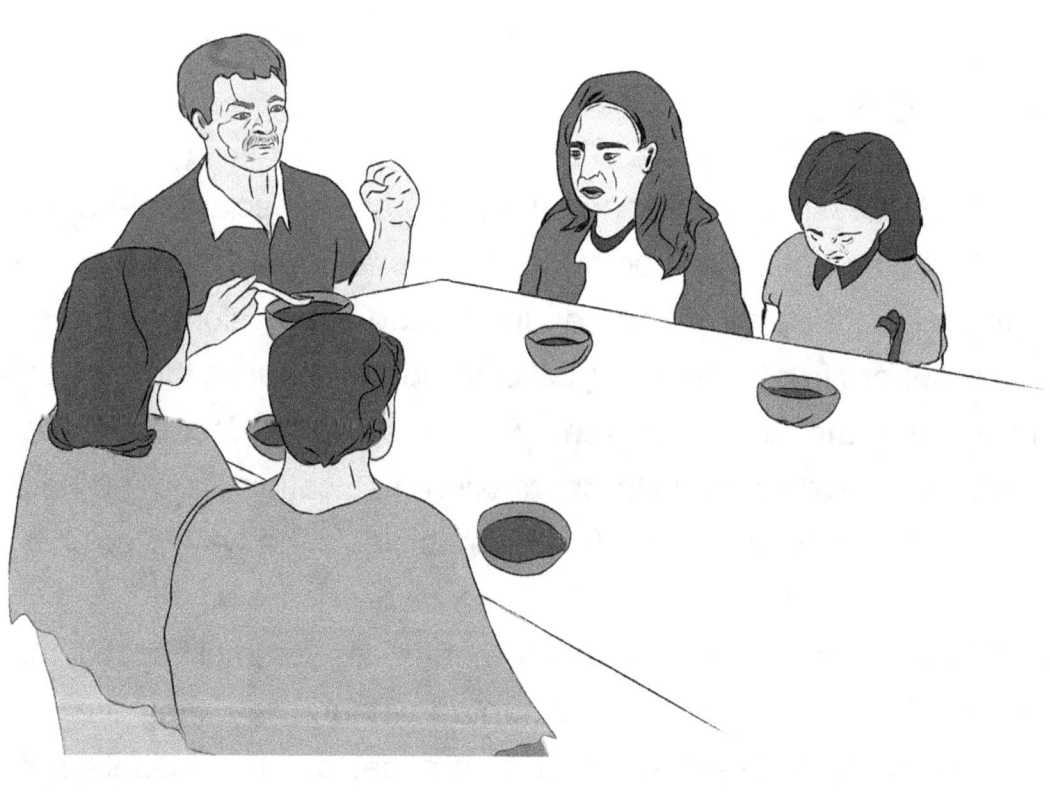

Case Twenty-Two

The Angry Middle Eastern Father

On a very busy day, my next appointment was with a large family of five, the Imams. In his request for an appointment, the oldest son said that they didn't know what was wrong with their father. I made a point of walking out to the waiting room to invite them to my office. It didn't have seats for five, so the secretary had to bring in two seats. Soon everyone was seated, with the father, guided by his son, sitting next to me. Mr. Imam was a 64-year-old man who looked healthy with a big mustache. I looked at him and asked what brought the family in today. (Working with families, I always direct my first question to the identified patient.) His answer surprised me. "I have no idea, ask them," he said. He paused. I felt he wanted to add something, so I waited before directing questions to the rest of the family. He looked at me and said, in a monotone: "No one listens to me anymore". He stopped right there. I could now begin asking questions to other family members. Next to Mr. Imam sat his wife, then his older daughter. The younger daughter and the son - the oldest child – were seated on the chairs that had been brought in.

I looked around to see who was ready to speak next. Everyone looked at the son. He seemed to be the family spokesperson. So, I asked if he could fill me in on what was going on. He began by saying that he was not sure but for the last two months his dad had become angry and very loud, pounding on the table, and shouting if any request of his was not carried out immediately. He was even cursing, which was completely out of character for him. At this, Ms.

Imam began sobbing, comforted by the daughter next to her. I offered a tissue and paused the interview until Ms. Imam had regained her composure. She then said in Arabic (which happens to be my mother tongue) "We love him, and we will never want to not listen or disobey him. He is all we have got". At this, the younger daughter began sobbing. This was a close family indeed, yet the room was tense. Again, I paused and said reassuringly that we would get to the bottom of this and that I would do everything possible to be of help.

I looked back at the spokesman-son hoping for more details. He began by telling the story of how his family had fared since arriving from Syria in the late seventies. They had prospered. The father was a hard-working man with a stable job as an accountant, and a good provider who loved his family. And his family clearly revered him in turn. This prompted several questions for me. When did the anger bouts begin? Did they appear suddenly or gradually? Had anything significant preceded them?

The son answered me, but only indirectly. He first repeated that no one in the family would ever disobey or fail to carry out Mr. Imam's wishes. "Even after he retired," he added, "our respect for him never changed. He is our guide in life and we want him back as he was before the stroke!".

The stroke? I asked a touch flabbergasted. "When was the stroke? What kind of stroke was it and how bad?" No one was informed of these matters. I asked the son if he had brought with them the paperwork from the hospital: the Discharge Summary that outlines the reason for admission, identifies all tests performed and their results, and finally, all medications and follow-up plans. The son looked at me and asked in all sincerity if I thought the stroke could have anything to do with his father's issue. He insisted that upon discharge they had been reassured that their father was *fully recovered*. He then said that many family members (with good educations!) believed that his retirement and his stroke had combined to make him *depressed*. Depression, he believed was the reason for his anger. On this everyone nodded in agreement. And help with depression was what they expected from a psychiatrist.

Just now the father looked up and shouted, "I am *not* depressed! I keep telling you that. No one listens to me; I'm fed up". While he spoke in a loud voice, he did not look or even *sound* angry. Neither his *tone* of voice nor his facial expression conveyed anger. This brought to my mind a specific neurological condition, but I needed to put my intuition to a test. And first, to rule out depression, I turned to the father and asked him a series of diagnostic questions about depression. He said no to all of them. He said he had been sleeping well. (Despite having to visit the bathroom once or twice at night, he quickly fell asleep on returning to bed.) Ms. Imam confirmed his answers. His appetite had not changed; it was good. He never spoke of wanting to die or harming himself. (Suicide ideations go against Middle Eastern values and so would have been a major depression indicator.) I did not feel he was depressed either, although his monotone and expressionless face were striking features that needed explanation. I asked the son to bring me all medical records from the stroke hospitalization, particularly the actual MRI images, not just the report. He agreed to do so. They all left, apparently satisfied that I had definite ideas about how to help the father. I was hoping that my neurological intuition would prove correct.

Three days later, the son stopped by with the hospital records, including the MRI. They indicated that Mr. Imam had appeared at the hospital reporting a sudden weakness in his left arm. The weakness was moderate. His arm's sensation was also affected. But soon after admission, his arm had begun regaining both strength and sensation thanks to a program of physical therapy. The MRI confirmed my intuition: it revealed a relatively small lesion in the lower part of the right frontal lobe area. This abnormality is exactly what I expected and now it was time to confirm my clinical suspicion in the presence of the family.

But first, let me explain. If this damage had been on the left (or dominant side of the brain, in most people), the patient would have been suffering from what is called "aphasia," or difficulty with speaking. Aphasia comes in three primary varieties: *receptive* (cannot understand what is being said), *expressive* or *motor* (cannot say what they want to say), and *conductive* (cannot repeat what they just heard). But when the damage occurs on the right (or non-dominant side, in most people), the resulting deficit centers on voice intonations and emotions conveyed in speech and facial expressions. This problem comes in two major varieties; *receptive* (sufferers cannot decipher emotions in other people's speech or facial expressions), or *expressive* (their own speech becomes monotonic and without facial expressions). The right-side condition is called *Aprosodia*. In Mr. Imam's case, it was most likely of the motor or expressive variety.

It was now my task to test for Aprosodia. The clinical test is simple. I ask the patient to identify the tone of voice (e.g., happy, sad, angry, surprised, or inquisitive) in which you say a sentence (it is important that the words in the sentence do not by themselves indicate the emotion like "I am going to the movies"). The emotion embedded in the sentence must be indicated only by the tone of voice or facial expression. I usually start with a happy tone. Over the years I have often practiced the test on medical students and colleagues. None have ever had difficulty naming the emotion I was conveying in my sentence. If a patient correctly identifies the correct emotional tones of my sentences, I then ask the patient to repeat the sentence in the appropriate tone (i.e., happy, sad, angry, surprised, or inquisitive). This request is a no-brainer for almost everyone ranging from four-year-old children to seniors in their 90s. But would Mr. Imam pass it?

I started by testing first for the *receptive* variant. The family was now present. Mr. Imam had no trouble correctly identifying my happy tone of voice. For that matter, he accurately identified the tones when I repeated the sentence in angry, inquisitive, sad or surprised manners. He acted as if this was a silly exercise. I then asked him to repeat the same sentence in a happy voice. He did his best. But to everyone's amazement, he did not sound at all happy. I then asked him to repeat the sentence in a sad tone of voice. He sounded exactly the same as his first response. It was an absolute, flat, monotone.

Now came the most important question. I asked him to repeat the sentence and *sound angry*. Again, to everyone's surprise, he spoke in the same monotone, and with no sign of anger on his face. His responses to my additional requests that he shows surprise and inquisitiveness were equally flat. I informed Mr. Imam and his family that he suffered from a relatively mild instance of a neurological disability called *expressive aprosodia*. He and his family had just witnessed confirmation of this diagnosis.

I then explained things to the family. It was quite understandable that they could not hear his protests that no one was responsive to him anymore. His protests sounded hollow to everyone and unserious! The wife and children could now see why Mr. Imam had no other recourse but to shout (the loudness of his voice being unaffected) and do things like pounding on the table. Hearing my explanation of all this, the two daughters first began to comprehend their father's plight, then the son and the mother.

The son then asked the right question: how they could help their father? The answer was simple. Making eye contact with everyone, I told them that they should simply pay very close attention to Mr. Imam's *words*: not his tone of voice or his facial expression. I added that in time the control of his facial expressions should improve and perhaps recover fully, like his motor and sensory functions.

The family members left my office relieved by my diagnosis and encouraged by my favorable prognosis for Mr. Imam. I would see everyone again in three months. But a week before that appointment, the son called to inform me that his father was doing very well, and they no longer needed the appointment. Very glad indeed to hear the good news, I wished everyone the best of luck, and this case was complete.

My Thoughts:

The clinical concept of a "Differential Diagnosis" requires clinicians in all branches of medicine to develop complete lists of all possible causes for presenting symptoms. These lists are vitally important because factors of all kinds can create similarities in symptoms that make the correct diagnosis and proper treatment more difficult.

The importance of Differential Diagnosis is seen in the scenario of a psychiatrist being examined for board certification. If (s)he fails to produce a differential diagnostic list, whether for a simulated or a live patient, he will surely fail the exam no matter how clear-cut the case before her/him may be.

Now consider a person who complains of hearing voices, or auditory hallucinations. The first thought that occurs to most psychiatrists is schizophrenia. But hearing voices can have many other causes, including psychostimulants or hallucinogenic drug use, epilepsy, or even a brain tumor. A proper Differential Diagnosis list for hearing voices will include all possible causes. And it will state reasons for ruling out as many possible causes before narrowing the diagnostic possibilities down to one or more *probable* causes.

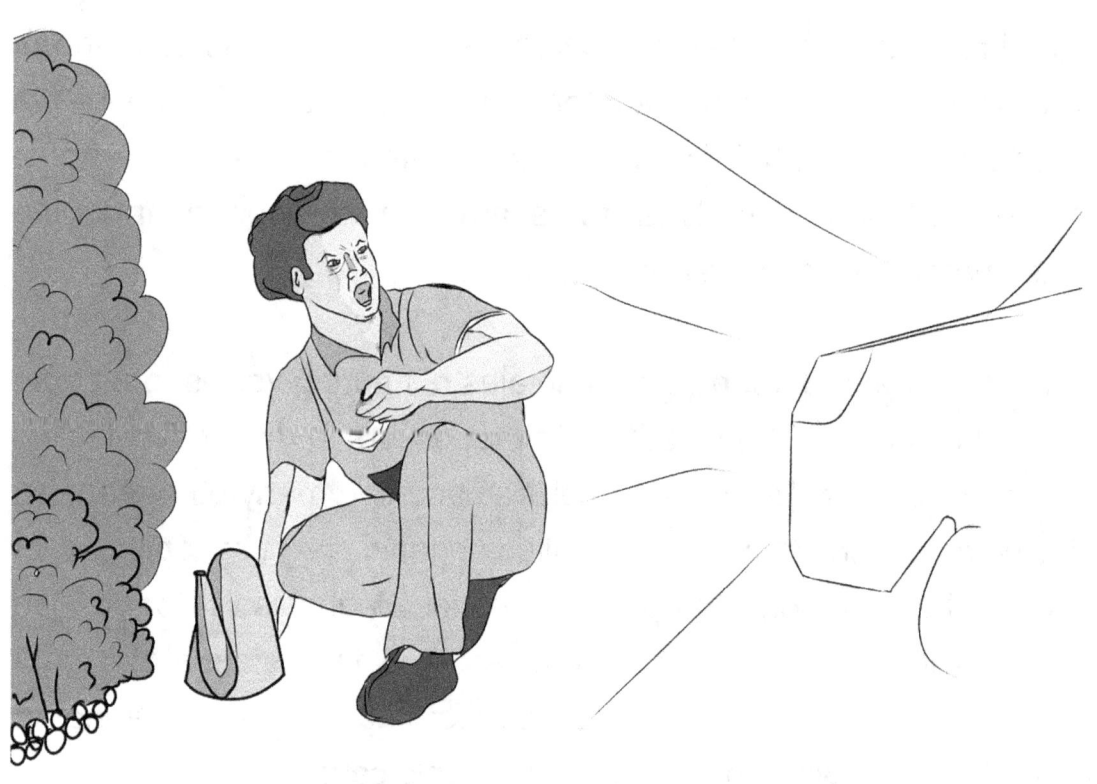

Case Twenty-Three
The Story of the Amnestic Killer

Mr. Wagner, a single 32-year-old man who used to be employed as a clerk, was now residing in a long-term psychiatric facility. He had murdered a woman but was completely *amnestic* – unable to remember anything - about the details of his crime. At trial, it had been revealed that he was under the influence of mind-altering drugs at the time. At the facility, however, Mr. Wagner had long been a model patient who presented no abnormal behaviors. After several years of being fully cooperative with staff and on good terms with patients, he has been permitted to perform chores in the vast backyard of the hospital grounds, unsupervised.

One day, as he was gardening near the long, winding driveway that led to the hospital, a speeding car veered off the road and struck him. He was in a coma for a full week. As he began to awaken, he was heard screaming "No, no…." in a voice of utter horror. Then, in the presence of nurses and physicians, he began reliving and describing the details of his crime. He gave details that have not been revealed in court.

An EEG, that I interpreted/evaluated, revealed active epileptic activity in the temporal/hippocampal memory-related region.

My interpretation of the clinical developments was that Mr. Wagner's protective brain mechanisms, up until the time he was struck by the car, had been able to suppress a memory already weakened by the presence of the mind-altering drugs. But the strength of the epileptic activity emanating from the memory-related regions of his brain seems to have overpowered his brain's protective mechanisms, thereby allowing for the details of his crime to re-emerge in all their horror.

But that was not all. Once these suppressed memories made their way to Mr. Wagner's conscious awareness, they became a recurrent nightmare. They would not let him be. He had flashbacks during the day and nightmares at night. We medicated him with an antiseizure medication of the kind that has proven effective in managing bipolar disorders. Mr. Wagner's seizures subsided, and his nightmares became occasional.

My Thoughts:

While the presence of epileptic activity in the brains of some psychiatric patients has long been known and well-documented, the phenomenon continues to be largely ignored by psychiatrists and denied by neurologists. I have written extensively on this issue, notably in the journal *EEG and Clinical Neurosciences,* which dedicated a full issue to this topic (Boutros NN, 2009).

Summing up: the presence of an epileptic discharge does not mean that the patient is suffering from epilepsy (Shelley et al, 2008). In my view, this discharge merely suggests a higher level of excitability (i.e., hyper-responsiveness) in the brain tissue where the activity is detected. In cases where this brain tissue is related to a given behavior, then that behavior is likely to manifest as abnormal. In such cases, therapy may not correct the aberrant behavior, and a medication that normalized the abnormal excitability would be expected to help. The only way to detect this kind of activity is by performing an EEG, which is widely available and relatively inexpensive.

I would add that psychiatrists often use anti-seizure medications to treat many psychiatric conditions without a solid rationale. But EEG testing can go far in providing an accurate rationale for the use of these medications. EEG testing can also help establish a more accurate diagnosis, thereby informing a patient's long-term care management.

To summarize the experience of my 40 years of clinical practice: EEGs can be the most helpful in situations where an individual

- has developed psychiatric symptoms at an unusually advanced age or in an unusual fashion, such as in the accident that befell Mr. Wagner
- has suffered repeated aggressive episodes, panic attacks, and/or dissociative symptoms (i.e., time lapses when the patient does not know what happened during this time). (Boutros et al, 2014a; 2014b).

Furthermore, for autistic children, EEG testing can reveal unsuspected epileptic activity in a small percentage of children (Swatzyna et al, 2018). The presence of such may prove invaluable in informing the child's treatment.

Finally, my neurology colleagues and I have been able to show that the presence of epileptic activity in the absence of seizures in a group of laboratory rats does significantly affect their behavior (Barkmeier et al, 2012). This topic, with ramifications, is discussed in two books of mine (Boutros et al, 2011; Boutros NN, 2014)

References:

Barkmeier DT, Senador D, Leclercq K, Pai D, Hua J, Boutros NN, Kaminski RM, Loeb JA. "Electrical, Molecular and Behavioral Effects of Interictal Spiking in the Rat," *Neurobiology of Disease* 47(1): 92-101, 2012

Boutros NN. Inter-ictal Spikes in Psychiatric Patients: A Controversy in Need for Resurrection." *Clinical EEG and Neuroscience*: Special Issue: "The Interictal Spike: What does it mean?," 40(4): 239-244, 2009

Boutros NN, Ghosh S, Khan A, Bowyer SM, Galloway MP. "Anticonvulsant Medications for Panic Disorder: A Review and Synthesis of the Evidence," *International Journal of Clinical Psychiatry in Practice*. 18(1):2-10, 2014a

Boutros NN, Kirollos SB, Pogarell O, Gallinat J. "Predictive Value of Isolated Epileptiform Discharges for a Favorable Therapeutic Response to Antiepileptic Drugs in Non-epileptic Psychiatric Patients," Journal of Clinical Neurophysiology 31(1): 21-30, 2014b

Shelley BP, Trimble MR, Boutros, NN. "Electroencephalographic Cerebral Dysrhythmic Abnormalities in the Trinity of Nonepileptic General Population, Neuropsychiatric, and Neurobehavioral Disorders," *Journal of Neuropsychiatry and Clinical Neurosciences* 20(1): 7-22, 2008

Swatzyna RJ, Boutros NN, Genovese AC, MacInerney EK, Roark AJ, Kozlowski GP. "Electroencephalogram (EEG) for Children with Autism Spectrum Disorder: Evidential Considerations for Routine Screening," *European Journal of Child and Adolescent Psychiatry*, 2018 Sep 14. PMID: 30218395

Boutros NN, Galderisi S, Pogarell O, Riggio S. *Electroencephalography in Clinical Psychiatry*, Wiley-Blackwell, Hoboken, NJ, 2011. ISBN 9780470747827

Boutros NN, *Standard EEG: A Research Roadmap for Neuropsychiatry*. Springer, 2014

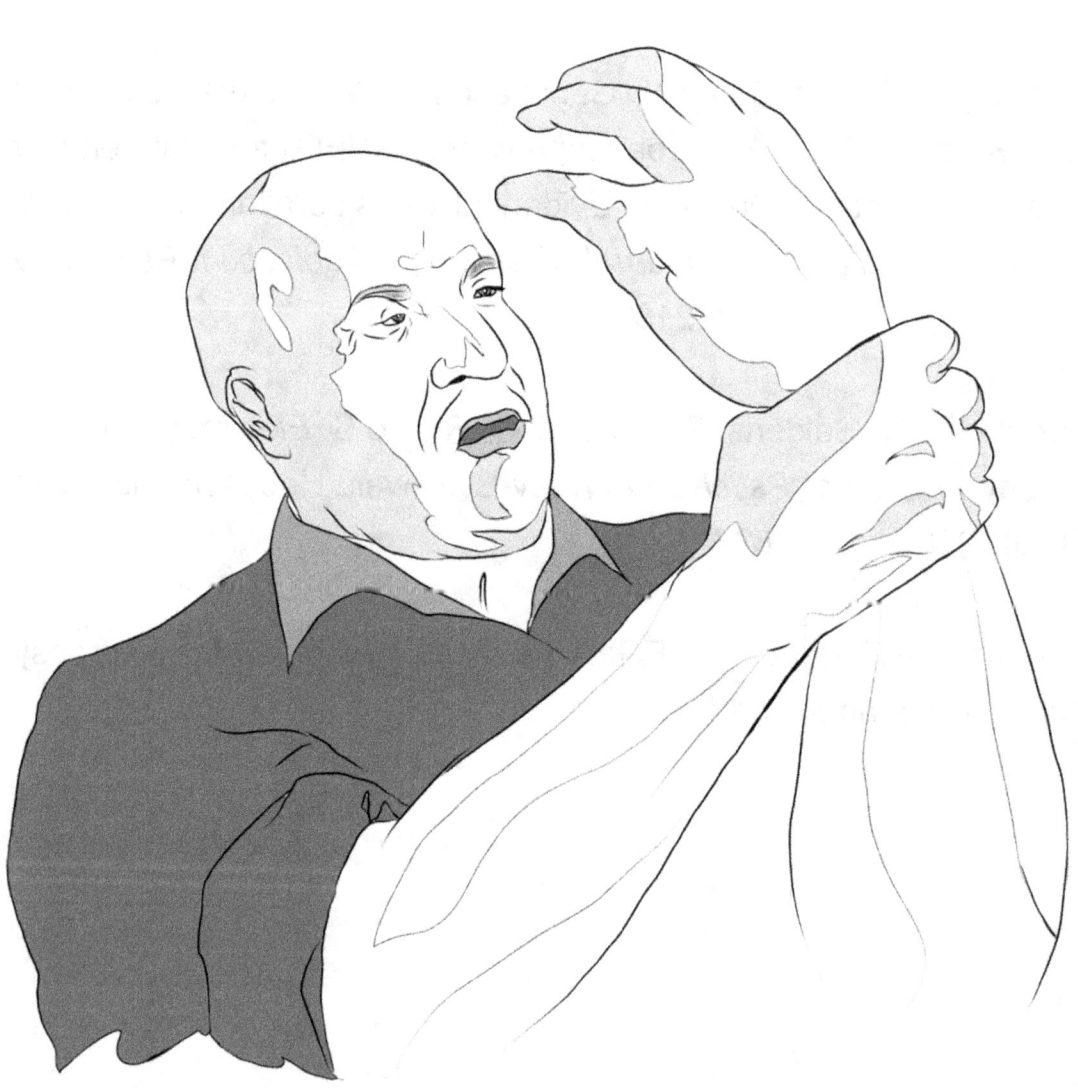

Case Twenty-Four
The Unruly Hand

Mr. Udell, a Londoner living in the United States, was 42 years of age, married, and the father of two healthy boys. For some twelve years, he had been successful as an insurance salesperson. But he was a chain smoker. He had attempted to quit several times but to no avail. In addition, he had a strong family history of high blood pressure and elevated blood cholesterol. He was in the upper range of his ideal weight. The only exercise he had was a fair amount of walking required by his work as a salesman.

His life seemed to be going smoothly, without major issues. But one day, with nothing unusual going on, he unthinkingly picked up an expensive shoe at a department store and placed it in his shopping cart. At the checkout, he was surprised to see the shoe in his cart and promptly returned it with an apology. He forgot the matter, not thinking even to tell his wife about it. A few days later he was in a grocery store, again with a shopping cart. Again, without thinking, he grabbed a bar of his favorite pistachio chocolate and placed it in his pocket. But this time a security guard spotted him, and police met him at the check-out. Again Mr. Udell had no memory of the incident. He paid for the chocolate, apologized, and was allowed to return home. This time he told his wife about the matter. She was as perplexed as he; behavior like this was completely out of character. After talking things over, they decided that she would join him on future shopping trips. She noticed that the left hand twitched occasionally but nothing more serious happened. She assumed that it must be some form of nervousness and he agreed.

But one day Mr. Udell had to take the subway to work. The train was crowded, and without knowing it, he stood next to a female passenger. Unbeknownst to him, his left hand reached out and touched her very inappropriately. She screamed and angrily insisted on reporting the incident to the police. He was taken in. Visited by his wife, they realized that this was a continuation of the two previous incidents – all three carried out by Mr. Udell's left hand!!

The next morning, before a judge, Ms. Udell insisted that these incidents were completely out of character for her husband of 20 years. The judge, noting that Mr. Udell had no prior criminal record and had long been gainfully employed, agreed with Ms. Udell and ordered him to be seen by a psychiatrist right away and to report back to court in six weeks. Ms. Odell called the psychiatry department at the university medical center where I was running a Neuropsychiatry clinic.

Her call came first to the outpatient department. The alert outpatient secretary decided to inform the Department Chairperson about this unusual case. The chairperson, sensing a possible brain (not psychiatric) issue at play here, asked me to do a workup on Mr. Udell first before sending him to a psychiatrist.

Mr. and Ms. Udell appeared at my office at the appointed time. From the moment he walked in it was obvious that he was exhibiting the classic signs of Alien Hand Syndrome. The poor man's left hand was literally tied to his left pants pocket. And it was with difficulty that Mr. Udell, using his right hand, was keeping his left hand from breaking loose. Both he and Ms. Udell were embarrassed, to say the least, and it took me some time before I could make them feel more relaxed and at ease.

Fortunately, Mr. Udell's predicament had a clear explanation in neuroscience. It begins with the fact that a stroke can damage or even sever the connection between the two hemispheric frontal lobes. When this happens, the right motor control systems (which control the actions of the left hand) will no longer be under the control of the dominant left hemisphere motor control apparatus. In this case, the left hand will no longer be under the usual control of the conscious brain. It may start acting out, so to speak, entirely on its own, in any number of bizarre ways ranging from compulsively pushing lots of elevator buttons (like a child) or shoplifting or touching inappropriately, as in the case of Mr. Udell.

So far, so good. But Mr. Udell had no history of a stroke. None, at least, that the patient or his wife were aware of. But I recalled his many risk factors for stroke: high blood pressure, chain smoking, and lack of vigorous exercise. So, I ordered a brain MRI. Three days later, the results showed that Mr. Udell had suffered a small stroke that affected the region mentioned above, causing this strange syndrome.

Obviously, such actions by a person with an Alien-Hand-Syndrome cannot be said to have been *willed* by that person. Sadly, my patients suffering from this syndrome all reported that the only way to prevent these bizarre acts was to tie the left hand into their pockets before leaving home. Even then, they would feel the offending arm squirming and trying to free itself. Unfortunately, there is at present no accepted treatment for this condition, except the possibility that the brain has sometimes been known to heal itself over time. If you have seen the classic 1964 comedy/drama Dr. Strangelove, you will probably recall seeing Peter Sellers, as Dr. Strangelove, struggling with his left hand to suppress the Heil Hitler salute.

The correct identification of Mr. Udell's affliction along with the explanation I gave of it in court sufficed for the judge to dismiss the case against M. Udell, and for the company to keep him on the job. He simply had to remember to tie his left hand down before leaving his house. Six months later, the problem was still with him at follow-ups, albeit at a much less intrusive and bothersome level.

My Thoughts:

It seems like eons ago, but the fact is that just a few decades ago the two clinical fields of Psychiatry and Neurology were seen as parts of a single discipline. The advent of Psychoanalysis caused the field of Psychiatry to move away from its previous commitment to being evidence-based. Freud (the father of Psychoanalysis) himself was a serious student of the brain in the earlier years of his career. Progressively the field of psychiatry lost interest in the brain as the seat of mental illness (brainless Psychiatry). At the same time, the field of Neurology, perhaps in reaction to the unempirical abstractions of psychiatry, decided to reject any concepts that were not empirically derived. This included even the time-honored concept of the human mind (Mindless Neurology).

But few academic departments of Psychiatry and Neurology are joint departments with a single chairperson. True, the certifying specialty board of both fields is the same: The American Board of Psychiatry and Neurology. *My experience persuades me that all medical disciplines dealing with the brain (i.e., Neurology, Neurosurgery, rehabilitation, and Psychiatry) should be housed in close proximity, if not in the same Clinical Neurosciences Department. Today, the need is pressing for cross-disciplinary interactions, which I am sure will benefit all fields and patients.*

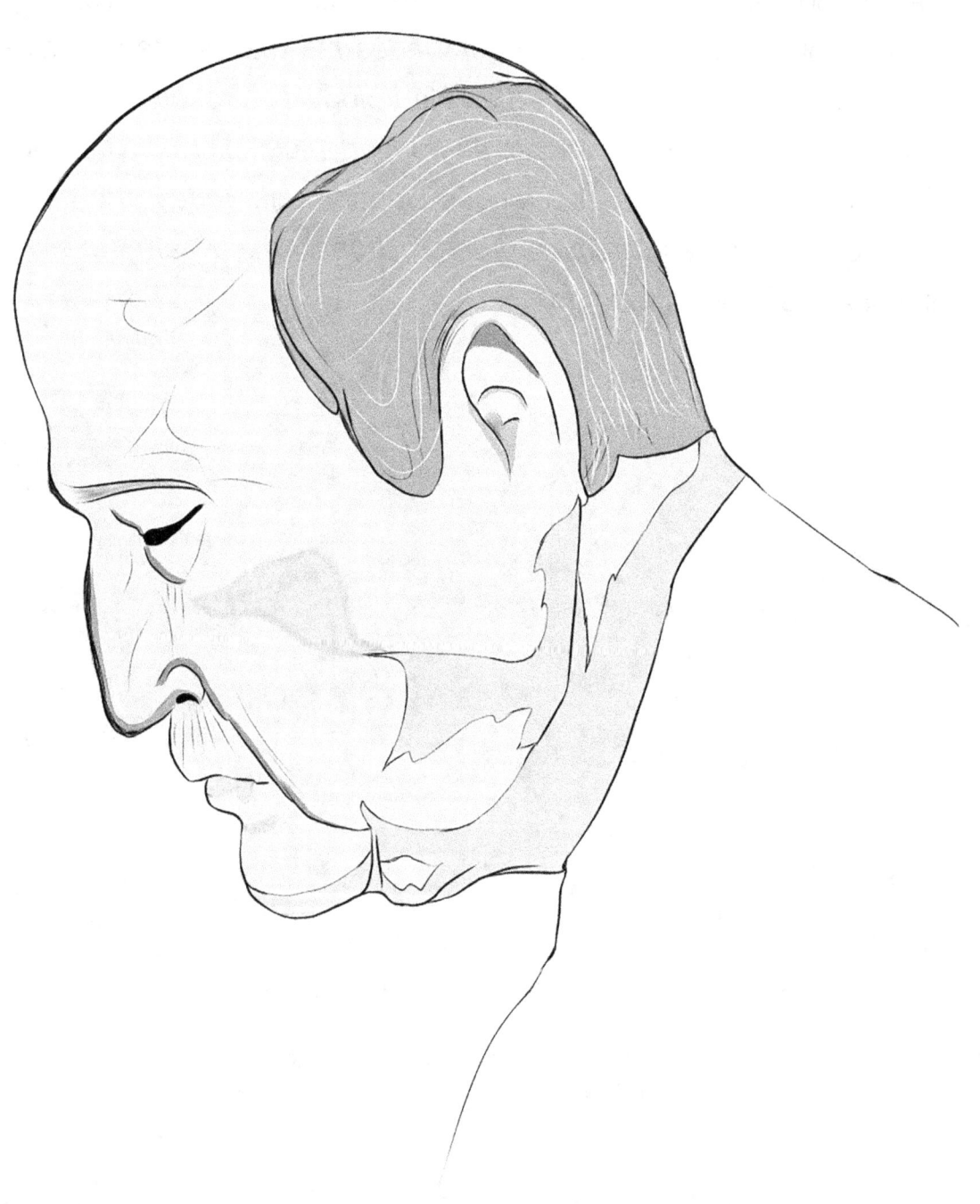

Case Twenty-Five
Depressed or Not Really?

Mr. Pfefferbaum was a 60-year-old married man and the father of four grown children. He had recently lost his job due to a massive layoff at his company. That said, he was well off financially and prepared to accept an earlier retirement than he had planned. He volunteered at his church and found several activities to occupy his time. But five months into his retirement, he suddenly lost the motivation to even get out of bed in the morning. He no longer wanted to go to church even though he knew the church depended on his active involvement on several committees, a few of which he had created himself. Understandably, his family members and friends attributed his sudden behavioral change to depression from being laid off from his job. His family decided to bring him to see a psychiatrist.

They made the appointment, and it was my turn to take the next patient. On the appointment date, Mr. Pfefferbaum was brought in by two of his children, both educated and successful businessmen. They stated simply that their father had become very depressed since his forced retirement. I started to interview the father who indeed looked very depressed. His spontaneous movement was decreased despite not having any motor limitations (a sign of depression called psychomotor retardation). I started by asking him how he felt. His answer was "absolutely fine Doctor." I was surprised. So, I began asking him about the symptoms of depression. His sleep was good, with no recent changes. So was his appetite, with no recent weight loss. Did he ever think of hurting himself or ending his life? To which he gave me a faint smile and said that the thought never crossed his mind. I turned to the two sons and asked if they ever saw their father crying. They both said "never." Now I was perplexed.

Although Mr. Pfefferbaum looked physically depressed, psychological signs of depression were missing. This combination put to mind the possibility of an affliction known as Pseudo Depression. It occurs in association with a brain lesion that affects the motivational centers of the brain. It makes the patient look physically depressed without suffering mental depression. Yet pseudo-depressed persons are not immune from developing depression as a complication of this disorder.

In Mr. Pfefferbaum's case, I concluded the patient was not suffering from a major Depressive Disorder. Suspecting a brain lesion resulting from a minor, previously undetected stroke, I ordered an MRI. Three days later the results confirmed a small lesion exactly where I thought it would be. I called the family, told them the good news (and news of a minor stroke was indeed good news in this case), and scheduled a time for them to see me again.

This time, Mr. Pfefferbaum was accompanied by three of his children. They were very curious about their father's condition. Mr. Pfefferbaum looked the same as the initial visit. I tried to ascertain just when the stroke had occurred but no one, including the patient himself, had the faintest memory of a possible stroke. I prescribed two medications: one for the standard management of a person at high risk of strokes, and the other an activating medication: a psychostimulant like those routinely used for ADHD and hypersomnia (when one is too sleepy). I explained to the family that an antidepressant, prescribed for depression, would be inappropriate in this case. Within a week, Mr. Pfefferbaum was no longer looking depressed. And he was busily involved in his church activities.

My Thoughts:

Here with Mr. Pfefferbaum's case, I renew my call for closer collaboration and even unification of the two fields of Psychiatry and Neurology. Their continued separation is harmful to the patients. At a minimum, the two fields – departments at each hospital or university - should hold joint Grand Rounds at least monthly to ensure that patients like Mr. Pfefferbaum are promptly and correctly diagnosed. In addition, I believe the time has come for Psychiatry and Neurology trainees to receive regular training in Neuropsychiatry. The field of Neuropsychiatry is now well established, with a good number of textbooks covering the discipline. There also exist a good number of fellowship training programs to enable both psychiatrists and neurologists to specialize in managing patients who fall into the grey area that separates the two disciplines.

I have long been concerned about the absence of objective laboratory tests for psychiatric disorders, including Major Depression. Mr. Pfefferbaum's case was an instance of the need for these tests: the man looked and acted depressed but was not suffering from a Major Depressive Disorder. Quite likely, a general practitioner or an unwary psychiatrist would have prescribed antidepressant medications. While the newer generation of antidepressant medications is safe, the resulting delay in the accurate diagnosis of a neurological condition would only prolong the patient's suffering. As I mentioned in Case # eight (Mr. Raoul), the existence of an abnormal pattern of rapid eye movement in the REM stage of sleep could serve as the basis of a diagnostic test for Major Depression (Arfken et al, 2014). Similarly, as I mentioned in case # 21 (Ms. Daniels), the Dexamethasone suppression test is a fairly reliable indicator of Major Depression (Mokhtari et al, 2013). It remains to be seen whether the combination of these two tests would be an advance, over mere clinical impressions, in diagnosing Major Depression.

References:

Arfken CL, Joseph A, Sandhu GR, Rhoers T, Douglass AB, Boutros NN. "The status of sleep abnormalities as a diagnostic test for major depressive disorder," *Journal of Affective Disorders*, 156;36-45, 2014.

Mokhtari M, Arfken C, Boutros NN. "The DEX/CRH Test for Major Depression: a Potentially Useful Diagnostic Test. *Psychiatry Research*, 30; 208 (2): 131-9, 2013.

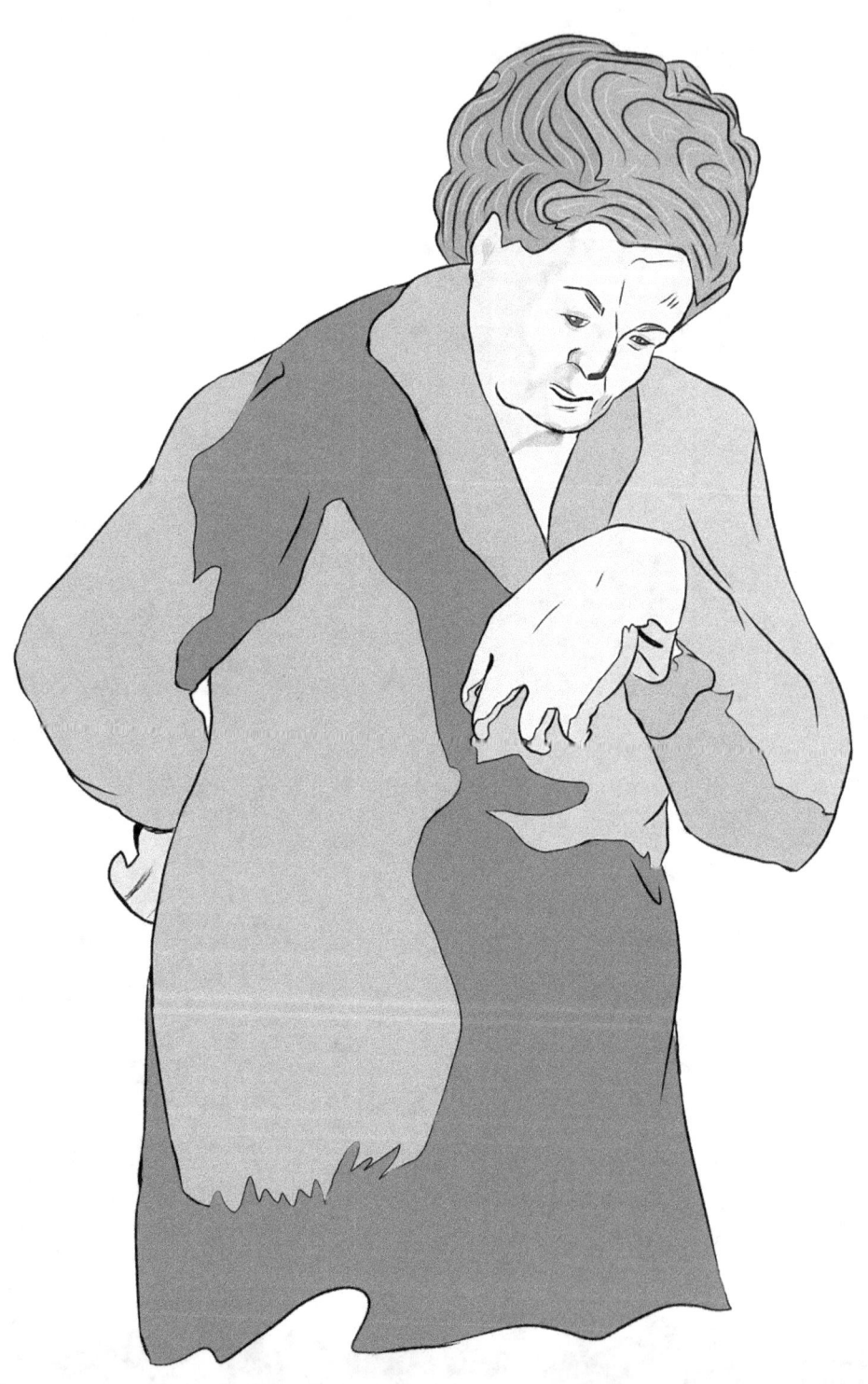

Case Twenty-Six

Condemned to Die from a Disease She Did Not Have!

Hanna was a 42-year-old woman, married and the mother of one daughter, Paula. She was referred to my Neuropsychiatry clinic from the Movement Disorder Program of the Neurology Department. The reason given for the referral by the movement disorders specialist was that he suspected she did not have an actual movement disorder – Huntington's Disease – and that her problem was "all in her head". Earlier in this book, I discussed cases when patients present with an apparent neurological disorder that lacks the needed evidence of brain pathology. And in such cases, the proper diagnosis can be Conversion Disorder. While actual mechanisms that produce these symptoms are not yet well understood, available research strongly suggests brain abnormalities of some kind.

Hanna showed up at my office on time accompanied by Paula, who was in her early twenties. Hanna was literally writhing as she walked in, a strange and concerning sight. Mother and daughter were equally anxious. Hanna immediately declared that she did not understand why she was being sent to a "shrink." She said "Doctor, my mother, and her mother both died of this," and said in a tone of voice that told me she thought she was soon going to die of it too: "it" being the dreaded Huntington's disease.

At the time I saw Hanna, effective treatments for Huntington's Disease did not exist, and the disease, as a result, was effectively a death sentence. With it, the patient usually deteriorates and dies within a few years. It was a terrifying diagnosis then and remains so today, despite the development of partial treatments.

Then Paula volunteered that her mother had gotten much worse over the last couple of years. They were now thinking of traveling to the Mayo Clinic for a definitive diagnosis and proper care. Hanna added that she not only could no longer "take care of Paula" but also had become a burden on her. This added a whole new dimension to the conversation. And though I could understand her, Hanna was having difficulty with her speech as well.

I asked if they had brought any medical records detailing tests performed to date. They were surprised – with reason – that I did not already have these records. I picked up the phone and got someone to overnight Hanna's records to me. I then completed my examination of Hanna, focusing on depression and possible suicidal tendencies. On this point, she acknowledged some self-destructive thoughts, but these struck me as not imminent. Seeing no immediate danger, I scheduled them for a return appointment the following week.

The next morning, I received the requested records. Reviewing them, it was obvious that the Movement Disorder specialist had spared no effort in attempting to make an accurate diagnosis. Her MRI picture of the brain revealed no abnormalities. Genetic testing as well was negative. At this point, I did not see the need for a trip to the Mayo Clinic, and I had reasons for recommending that treatment remain local. In my next appointment with Hanna and Paula, we discussed the test results at length. When Paula asked what

I thought was going on, I explained that the terrifying prospect of Huntington's Disease and the death of Hanna's mother and grandmother from this affliction had probably created in Hanna a severe anxiety leading to a Conversion Disorder: the conversion of a psychological fear to a set of physical symptoms that can mirror an affliction such as Huntington's Disorder. I carefully explained that Hanna's problem was by no means "all in her head." I said that I did not believe Hanna was suffering from the disease that killed her mother and grandmother, but that what she was going through felt excruciatingly real all the same.

"Is there a treatment," asked Paula. My answer was supportive and affirmative: a combination of medications to lower Hanna's anxiety and deal with her depressive symptoms, all combined with psychotherapy. Hanna seemed unconvinced, but Paula looked interested. I stated plainly that I did not see the need for a trip to the Mayo Clinic. They asked for time to think, and we scheduled a repeat visit in another week.

On the day of their visit, however, they called to cancel the appointment. A week later, I received a call from a neurologist at the Mayo Clinic who was seeing Hanna. I shared with him my views. The neurologist agreed with the conclusions of our local neurologist: that Hanna's issues were "all in the head"? Two weeks later Hanna and Paula were back in my office and prepared to commence the treatment I had proposed at our last visit.

Weekly psychotherapy and the prescribed medications worked slowly but progressively to decrease the level of Hanna's anxiety and, with it, the severity of her writhing movements and speech problems. After a year of treatment, and with my continued support and that of her psychotherapist, Hanna's symptoms had completely abated. And Hanna now welcomed the support of her daughter.

My Thoughts:

It is worth noting that the incidence of *psychiatric* complications in almost all movement disorders (e.g., Huntington's Disease, Parkinson's Disease, etc..) is elevated or exaggerated in comparison to comparably severe or disabling disorders. In Huntington patients, suicide is a real concern. A patient with Huntington's Disease can be suicidal while not being clinically depressed. Generally speaking, the more relaxed and stress-free a patient with a movement disorder is the less severe abnormal movements become. As if to confirm this, abnormal movements completely disappear while the patient is sleeping.

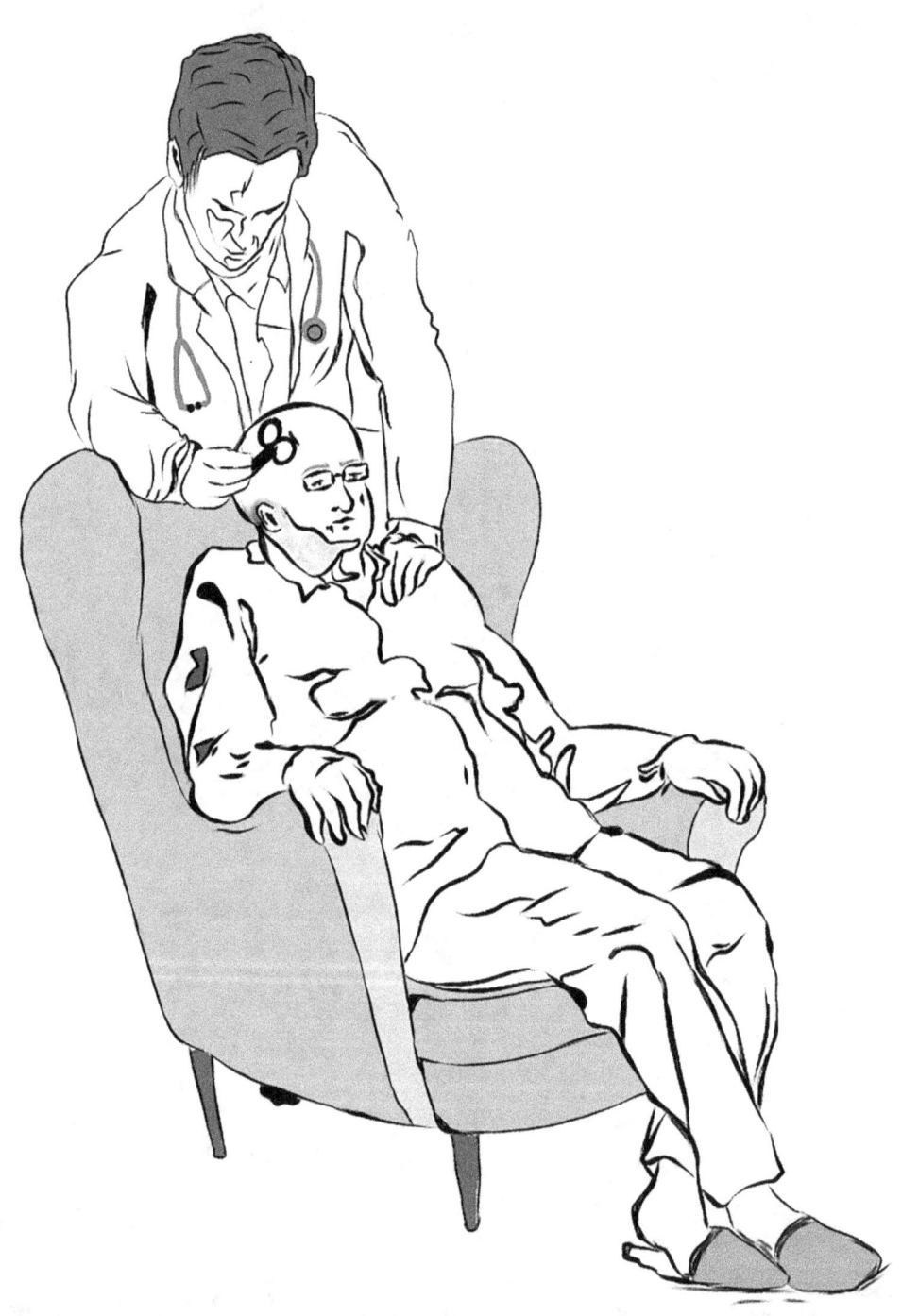

Case Twenty-Seven
The Power of Placebo

I was actively recruiting for one of my clinical research studies. I informed all clinicians in the medical community about the research project and the qualifications required for patients to enroll in it. This study would help to advance an emerging treatment method for depressed patients who had resisted both medication and psychotherapy. Where these traditional treatment methods had failed, the idea behind this new method was to help such patients by reactivating the sub-normally active frontal lobes of their brains. The technique was to direct a magnetic charge to these areas by means of a device that had accumulated a magnetic charge into a stimulation coil which, placed on the proper part of the patient's head, would be discharged into the brain at a specific frequency and at specific magnetic strengths. The procedure would be virtually pain-free. The technical name of the procedure is Transcranial Magnetic Stimulation (TMS).

Our study would compare the clinical therapeutic (or beneficial) effects of an *active* magnetic charge as opposed to a placebo consisting of a virtually *inactive* magnetic charge. To the test subjects, testing of active and inactive charges would look virtually identical. The difference between them would consist simply of the placement of the device. It would be placed flush with the targeted part of the brain in the active group by contrast with the sideways placement of the device with patients in the placebo group. This would ensure that all test subjects, the active group, and control group, had every reason to believe that they were receiving the active magnetic charge.

One morning I received a call from a clinician in town who was desperate to help one of his patients whom he said had been unresponsive to any form of treatment over a period of years. After answering a number of questions, he made it clear that his patient met all criteria for enrollment in our study, and an initial appointment for the first treatment session was set up.

An important component of my study would be the repeated post-treatment assessments of the severity of a patient's depression. This we would do using a standard measure called The Hamilton Depression Rating Scale (HDRS). Normally HDRS scores above 10 indicate some form of depression. But in order to qualify for this study, the patient had to score at least 20.

On the appointment date for the first session, the patient appeared on time. Mr. Trimble was a 50-year-old married father of two children. He had an advanced college degree and according to the paperwork that accompanied him, he was a successful businessman. His HDRS score of 32 placed him in the range of "severely depressed." His therapist's paperwork showed that Mr. Trimble had not responded to many months (almost two years) of intensive psychotherapy and despite having been placed on adequate doses of anti-depressant medication. At length, he was given a second medication that also failed to help. As a last resort, his psychiatrist prescribed a combination of medications which again got no good results.

At this point, the treating psychiatrist suggested Electro-Convulsive Therapy (ECT) but his patient rejected it due to possible effects on his memory. The referring physician, having heard about our ongoing TMS research study, suggested the study to Mr. Trimble. Feeling desperate, he readily agreed to undergo the trial fully aware that there was only a 50-50 chance that he would receive the active treatment. On the morning of the first session and after completing his evaluation and being accepted into the study, Mr. Trimble signed a consent form stating his 50/50 chance of being randomized into the sham/placebo arm of the project.

Once a patient's data was entered into the computer, it was the computer (not a clinician) that decided which arm of the research study a patient would be assigned to. Much to my dismay, the computer randomized Mr. Trimble to the sham/placebo arm of the study. That said, any patient randomized to the sham component of the study would subsequently be eligible to receive the active treatment, free of charge. I was the only person in the entire laboratory who possessed this piece of information. Both the patient and all laboratory employees were kept blinded to the mode of treatment, active or placebo. As the *sideways* placement of the device was a giveaway to which arm the patient was assigned, I had to be the only test giver. Personnel who performed the assessments (i.e., HDRS) were not allowed in the room during TMS administration.

For each patient, treatment sessions would occur three times a week for two weeks for a total of six sessions. I had enrolled the pre-required number of patients (10 in each arm), all of whom were as severely depressed as Mr. Trimble. Up to this point, I had seen no improvements in patients randomized to the sham/placebo arm of the study, while I was seeing either modest or significant improvements in not some, but all patients randomized into the active treatment arm. Things looked to be going well for the study!

But then things changed. To my amazement (and I confess my dismay), Mr. Trimble began to show signs of improvement. Strong signs. By his third session, his HDRS score had dropped from 32 to 20. And by his fifth, it had plummeted down to 7. He was now *below* 10: the minimal HDRS standard of depression! In his final session, he was thrilled with the study, and at the end, we said our goodbyes and I wished him the very best of luck.

I had good reason for my dismay. Because the positive response of just one control group (placebo) patient to the sham treatment had effectively invalidated the otherwise conclusive results of the entire study. The difference between the two groups was now rendered non-significant, or inconclusive in lay terms. In addition to my not understanding why Mr. Trimble's condition had improved so dramatically, his unaccountable improvement would impact the prospects for the future continuation of what to me was a truly promising project.

At any rate, I now had to inform Mr. Trimble's doctor that his patient had been randomized to the sham treatment and had definitely not received any active magnetic charges. Hearing this, the doctor could not accept that his patient recovered due to a mere placebo. He insisted that the magnetic treatment must have done something hugely beneficial for his patient.

I too could not believe that Mr. Trimble's seemingly miraculous improvement was due to a sham treatment. Could it be that some magnetic charges had somehow found their way to a brain that was unusually sensitive to their effects? But this was mere speculation.

I regret the inconclusive ending of this case study. But at least Mr. Trimble had recovered. I regret also that circumstances prevented me from finding out how long his recovery lasted.

My Thoughts:

Eventually a medical device manufacturer, perhaps responding to stories like this one, placed on the market a placebo device called the Sham-Coil, which emits no trace whatsoever of magnetic activity.

Some readers may ask why it is so important that a placebo arm be included in studies like this one. It is important because the power of persuasion suggestion can be so strong. And it is essential for researchers to confirm that any beneficial effects detected are due *only* to the medication (in this case, to the active charges) and not to the effects of merely *believing* in a treatment. It's for this reason that patients and testing clinicians alike must be kept ignorant as to whether patients are receiving active or placebo treatments.

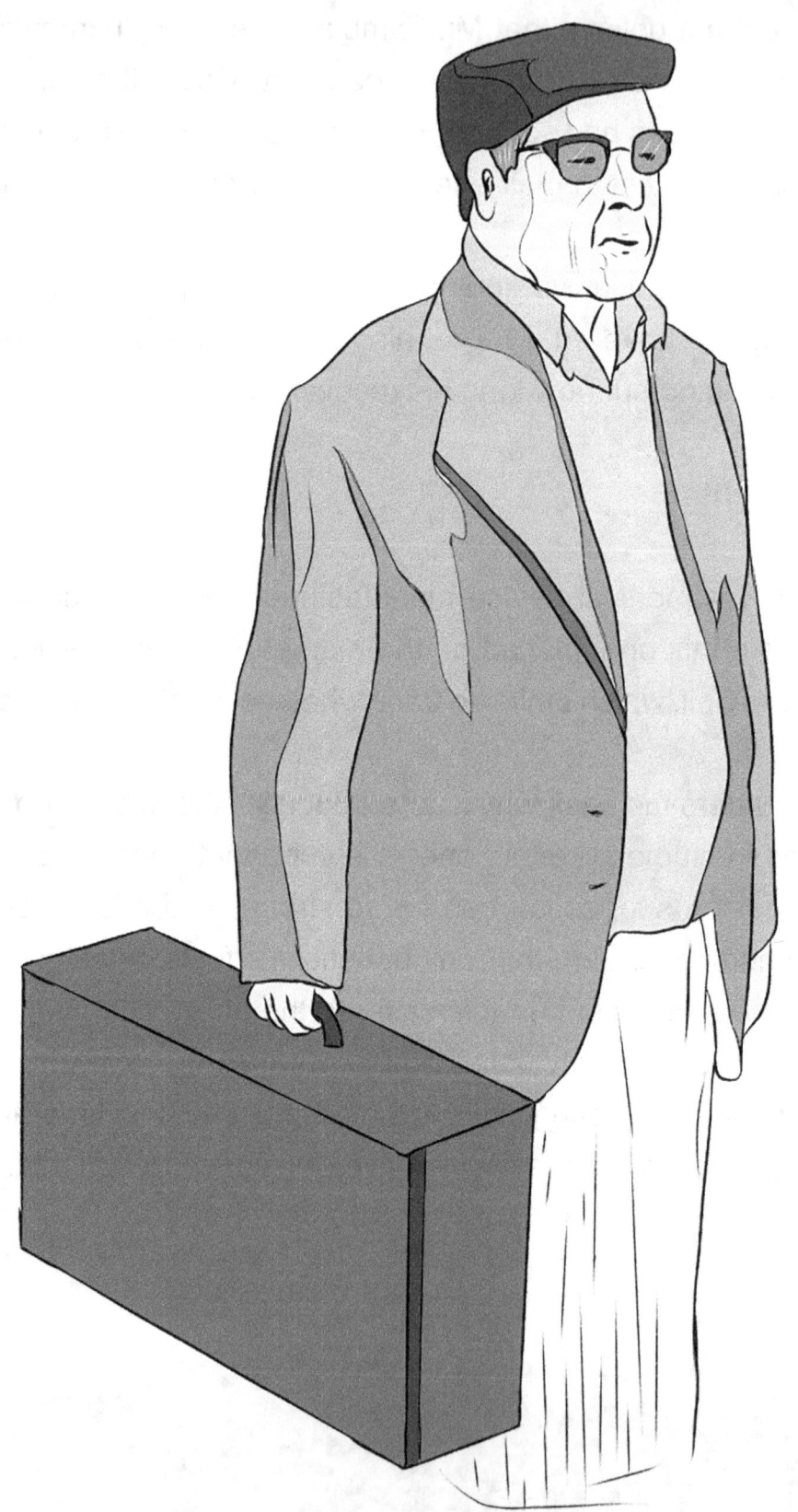

Case Twenty-Eight
The Prolific Writer

Mr. Tyler came to me via my regular Psychiatry Clinic after having waited three months for an initial evaluation. He was a single male of 34 years of age. The reason for the long delay was his insistence whenever he called my office that his need for an appointment was not urgent. On the appointment day, he showed up exactly on time. He was well-dressed and did not appear to be in any distress. I had no idea what had brought him to my clinic from the medical records he supplied. So, I started with the usual question: "What brings you to the clinic today?"

Mr. Tyler began by saying he wasn't sure I was the right person to help him. I encouraged him to just tell me what was going on. He started talking about his bad luck in life and how untrustworthy the people around him were. He said he was unable to maintain meaningful relationships, adding that "I thought it was only with the opposite sex, but I can't even make friends with my own sex." My next question was about his last romantic relationship. He said he had had several but none lasting more than a few months. The last one, about eight months ago, had lasted two months. Responding to my request for details, he volunteered that it had started well but because he had no steady job, his girlfriend ended up leaving him. He added that he felt doing so was not "Christian" of her.

I then inquired about his career. Since graduation from college at age 21 – some thirteen years earlier – Mr. Tyler had held just one job: as an accountant for five years. During this time, he had a stable romantic relationship that he hoped might lead to marriage. But then, he said, both his job and his romantic relationship deteriorated at the same time. He ended up with no friends, no relationships, and no job. He could not explain why, I now sense that something was very amiss with Mr. Tyler but was far from figuring it out. So, I asked some of my routine survey questions about the symptoms and signs of several possible psychiatric disorders in order to narrow down the possibilities.

Mr. Tyler basically denied any significant psychiatric symptomatology. He had no trouble sleeping, eating, focusing on his work, or being on time for appointments. He denied ever feeling depressed other than a "normal" dissatisfaction with a life situation like his. Never had he thought of hurting himself. He had no history of psychotic symptoms like hearing voices or imagining somebody plotting against him. He showed no symptoms of anxiety, such as apprehension or panic attacks.

The last two parts of my clinical evaluation usually inquire into personal and family medical histories, including psychiatric histories. Mr. Tyler indicated a family history of epilepsy and said that he himself had had a seizure while in college but was told by his college health service that it was insignificant. It went without treatment. He denied ever using illegal drugs or abusing prescription medications.

Time was now running short for our first session, and I had yet to begin to narrow down the possibilities of what was troubling Mr. Tyler. I wondered if his condition might be a long-term personality trait or disorder that might not be amenable to medical treatment and instead needs long-term psychotherapeutic treatment. At the end of the session, I asked Mr. Tyler to keep a diary of any significant happenings in his life, his moods, his sleep pattern, and his appetite until we met two weeks later.

Two weeks later he again showed up exactly on time, this time carrying a briefcase. Opening it, he brought out 35 pages of typed single-spaced writings. These, he said, were his notes and observations over the last two weeks, as I had requested. I could not read them during our 20-minute follow-up interview, but I did spend five minutes looking through them. The writing was rambling but clearly talked about how people did not care about him or even about the world. The very second page stated that people had gone away from God. I then asked Mr. Tyler to tell me more about the last two weeks. He spoke without interruption until the time was up. It was hard to terminate the session. He had spoken in a monotone but did not seem rushed or pressured, as I often see with patients in a manic state. Furthermore, while he clearly felt morally superior to those around him, his feelings did not amount to a delusion of grandeur. He gave no impression of thinking he was a profit, which would suggest being delusional!

My next session with Mr. Tyler ended with a diagnosis beginning to emerge. His family history of epilepsy, his history of a seizure, his prolific writing, and his moral superiority all pointed to the possibility that he was suffering from a brain disorder known as Temporal Lobe Personality Disorder (TLPD). I ordered an EEG and asked Mr. Tyler to return in two weeks, this time without asking him to keep a diary.

The EEG came back confirming my suspicion of epileptic activity in Mr. Tyler's temporal lobe. The activity was not severe enough to cause repeated seizures. But I was now considering the possibility of minor seizure manifestations that could well escape his notice. For our third session, Mr. Tyler again appeared on time and again with his briefcase. This time he handed me 40 more pages of single-spaced writing. Fortunately, between appointments, I had read his first 35 pages. These were hyper-religious and moralistic in tone. This time, I wasted no time inquiring about possible minor seizure manifestations. Indeed, he reported having had minor manifestations such as occasional staring for no reason or losing a period of time with no recall of what happened. It should also be noted that individuals with this syndrome tend to be hyposexual (uninterested in sex), which could contribute to their romantic difficulties.

I explained my theory that he might be suffering from Temporal Lobe Personality Disorder. We discussed his behaviors that are symptomatic of this diagnosis. I also explained his EEG findings. I now had to say that there is no known treatment for this condition. But then I suggested that monitoring and controlling his abnormal brain activity might help him in the long run. With his approval, I prescribed a seizure medication, known also to be psychoactive, which is often used to treat bipolar disorder. I emphasized that I did not think for a minute that he had bipolar disorder or major depression, and he agreed with this assessment.

During our now-monthly follow-ups, Mr. Tyler reported that he was taking his medication regularly. He reported that my explanation of TLPD has made him more keenly aware of his behavior and that he was making an effort not to be judgmental of others. This struck me as good progress

In our third follow-up appointment, four months into treatment, Mr. Tyler reported that his urge to write down all his ideas had decreased and that he had met a nice woman whom he was now seeing. He was also applying for jobs. This was very encouraging, and I supported his efforts and applauded his progress. In our fourth follow-up appointment, he reported having maintained his new relationship and landed a job. Follow-up a year later showed him to be holding both a steady job and a steady girlfriend while continuing the same medication.

A summary of a piece from *Scientific American*, March 2017.

In 1975 neurologists Stephen Waxman and Norman Geschwind, then both at Harvard University, published an analysis based on observations of their patients with temporal lobe epilepsy in which they reported that many of these patients had a tendency toward religiosity, intense emotions, detailed thoughts, and a compulsion to write or draw. This cluster of characteristics became known as the epileptic personality. Over the next decade, other researchers added hostility, aggression, lack of humor, atypical (usually reduced) sexuality, and obsessiveness to the list of personality traits supposedly associated with the condition.

By the 1980s, however, researchers began to question the notion of the epileptic personality altogether. They pointed out that the supposed core characteristics did not appear in all individuals with

temporal lobe epilepsy and that many also occurred in other patient populations. By the end of the 20th century, researchers came to a consensus that only a minority of temporal lobe epilepsy sufferers exhibited some of these core features.

My Thoughts:

Personality Disorders are uphill battles for any psychiatrist as there are no known medical treatments for them and the only known remedy is costly long-term psychotherapy, which lacks evidence of efficacy. Over the years, I personally developed the habit of rather bluntly presenting most of my patients suffering from a Personality Disorder with all or most of the evidence I had found of their symptoms. In fact, I would copy the symptom list from the DSM book and hand it to the patient with his or her symptoms simply checked off. Then we would talk. In my experience, this straightforward approach motivated many patients to change their images and behaviors as well.

Closing Remarks

Dear reader:

I sincerely hope that you found the above case histories both entertaining and informative. The choice of cases was based on their unusual nature and whether they convey a lesson to readers and clinicians. While not the main purpose of the book, the book, to some extent deals with the issue of stigma attached to psychiatric disorders. The issue of stigma is well known. Two main factors tend to be the major contributors to a disorder or a condition being stigmatizing. The first is attributing the problem to a personal characteristic that the person at some level is in control of, much like in sexually transmitted diseases. This is perhaps the major factor in the stigma associated with psychiatric disorders. A second factor is uncertainty regarding what the condition could lead to. The perception that the disorder is indicative of a character flaw leads to a reluctance to hire the person. The possibility of violence or the simple fear of lack of reliability could hinder an employer from offering a job to an otherwise qualified person. As you may have noticed, I avoided the term "mental Illness" throughout the book As I prefer the term "Psychiatric Disorders".

Efforts to deal with and combat the stigma associated with receiving a psychiatric diagnosis, or even just seeing a psychiatrist, are many but have had hardly any progress. The RECALCITRANT nature of the "mental" illness stigma will remain as long as the term "mental" remains. These disorders are stigmatizing because they are "mental" as opposed to regular physical disorders.

If we recall, for as long as its brain etiology, its biological cause, was unknown, "epilepsy" was a highly stigmatizing disorder. Suspected causes ranged from demonic possession to excessive masturbation. This is hardly the case now. Once the "biological" nature was fully and unequivocally identified, the disorder began to progressively lose its stigma. The stigma associated with epilepsy did not dissipate overnight and some level of stigma remains today. There is no reason to believe that the stigma associated with any psychiatric disorder will have a different fate. The stigma associated with tertiary neuro-syphilis- (general paresis of the insane or GPI) also did not dissipate except with the actual, almost, eradication of the disease itself, and that is likely because of its "morality" implications.

The full recognition of the biological nature of an illness will usher-in the beginning of the dissipation of the stigma. The realization of the biological nature of psychiatric disorders has come of age in the current era of "Biological Psychiatry". Progressively more psychiatrists describe themselves as Biological Psychiatrists. This term has come to mean that the psychiatrist relies heavily on medication (or biological treatments like TMS (case 27)). Biological psychiatrists continue to recognize the value of providing supportive therapy and educating patients and families about their illnesses. It is also argued throughout the book that the advent of laboratory-based objective diagnostic tests will also go a long way in dissipating stigma and helping patients seek help sooner and stick to the prescribed management. An interesting observation is that while the suicide rate among psychiatrists used to be the highest among MDs, the emergence of "Biological Psychiatry" was attended by a significant decrease in the suicide rate among psychiatrists. This change was attributed to the belief, during the Psychoanalysis dominated period, that a treatment failure was almost always a reflection on the competence of the psychiatrist whereas the advent of Biological Psychiatry underscored the significant lack of Knowledge about Psychiatric Disorders that underlies the common failure of available treatment. The guilt attended to treatment failures, being a common occurrence, has thus been alleviated.

One crucially important lesson I learned through my 50 years of teaching and taking care of patients, is that the practice of Psychiatry is both very easy and very difficult at the same time. Our mistakes whether diagnostic or therapeutic are very difficult to discover at least in the immediate or short term. This is unlike mistakes that can lead to endangering the lives of patients like taking a good kidney out by error!!! On the other hand, the ever-increasing volume of research in all sub-fields of Psychiatry makes it hard for the conscientious psychiatrist to keep up with advances in the field. A clinician must strive to be knowledgeable by constantly reviewing recent publications and attending the many national and international scientific conferences as his/her time allows. Clinicians must also be skeptical when approaching the diagnostic process and should avail themselves of any available diagnostic aids.

Finally, advocacy for psychiatric patients, particularly those with severe and persistent illnesses, is weak at best and frequently completely absent. This is an astonishing fact given that one out of every five humans suffers from psychiatric disorders of one form or another. It follows that it is almost impossible to live a life with never being exposed to psychiatric disorders by a friend or a relative. An effective organization representing this huge percentage of people could have immense lobbying power that would assure adequate and innovative care, legal protection of individuals incarcerated due to psychiatric disorders, and enough funding for research.

Currently one main organization advocates for "the mentally ill" in the US; the National Alliance for the Mentally Ill (NAMI). Several smaller organizations do as well. The World Health Organization advocates internationally and plays a bigger role in developing countries. Smaller organizations are focused on certain types of illnesses like schizophrenia, bipolar disorder, etc.

The term "Mental" embodies the duality of mind-brain or mental-physical. Doing away with this duality is our first step to burying stigma and relegating it to the history of medicine.

Acknowledgments

I would like to acknowledge the contributions of two individuals whose help made this book possible. Steve Sewall, Ph.D. for editing the book, and Anupam Sharma (Unquannu can be found on Fiverr) for the illustrations. I also acknowledge the constant and unwavering support of my wife, Sylvia, and my two children Tammer and Alexandria.

About The Author

Armed with enthusiasm and determination to pursue research in behavioral disorders and related neurosciences, I emigrated from Egypt to the USA in 1977 having attended medical school at Cairo University in Egypt. I had my first experience with psychiatry there. I completed training in psychiatry and neurology in Chicago, then pursued further specialized training in behavioral neurology and brain neurophysiology. All the training qualified me to understand the basic physiology of the brain and how that relates to behavior.

Much of what I learned helped me understand why people do what they do and, in some cases, believe in the most absurd ideas. I taught, conducted research, and practiced at the University of Texas (UT), Ohio State University (OSU), Yale University, Wayne State University (WSU), and the University of Missouri in Kansas City (UMKC). I also practiced and consulted in many private and state-operated facilities over the years. As a clinical scientist, I have been publishing extensively in national and international journals. I am fully aware of how facts can be presented and misrepresented, even in the most prestigious journals. This awareness influenced my writing of my seven scientific books, but more clearly in my book, "Humanist Psychiatry, both first and second editions" which is a hybrid scientific-popular book. I also published upward of 220 peer-reviewed scientific papers in national and international journals and contributed many chapters to several books over the years.

I completed my active medical career as the Chairperson of the Department of Psychiatry at the University of Missouri, Kansas City, and Director of the Behavioral Neurology Section of the Marion Block, Neuroscience Institute of the Saint Luke Medical Center in Kansas City. Currently, I continue to teach and mentor at RUSH University Medical Center in Chicago.

Other Books by the Author

Nash N Boutros. The Struggle Within. Amazon.com, 2022.

Nash N Boutros. A Journey from Orthodoxy to Humanism; We are not alone. Amazon.com, 2022.

Boutros NN. Humanist Psychiatry, 2nd edition. Nova Science Publishers. 2022. New York. ISBN: 978-1-68507-501-9

Clark DL, Boutros NN, Mendez FM. Brain and Behavior: An Introduction to Behavioral Neuroanatomy. Third Edition; Cambridge, Inc.ISBN-13978-0-52184050-7, 2010 (Translated into Spanish "El cerebro y la conducta; Neuroanatomia para psicologos" Manual Moderno, 2010.

Boutros NN, Galderisi S, Pogarell O, Riggio S. Electroencephalography in Clinical Psychiatry. Wiley-Blackwell, Hoboken, NJ, 2011. ISBN 9780470747827

Boutros NN (Ed). International Psychiatry and Behavioral Neurosciences, Yearbook Volume I. Nova Science Publishers. January 2011.

Boutros NN (Ed). International Psychiatry and Behavioral Neurosciences, Yearbook Volume II. Nova Science Publishers. January 2013; ISBN: 978-1-62257-566-4.

Boutros NN: Standard EEG: A Research Roadmap for Neuropsychiatry. Springer, 2014.

Psychophysiology in Psychiatry and Psychopharmacology' volume of "Current Topics in Behavioral Neurosciences'. Kumari V, **Boutros NN,** Bob P Editors. Current Topics in Behavioral Neurosciences" (Series Editors Profs. Charles Marsden, Bart Ellenbroek and Mark Geyer) provides critical and comprehensive discussions of the most significant areas of behavioral neuroscience research. Springer Publisher, 2014.

Clark DL, **Boutros NN,** Mendez FM. Brain and Behavior: An Introduction to Behavioral Neuroanatomy. Fourth Edition; Cambridge University Press, 2018. ISBN 978-1-316-64693-9

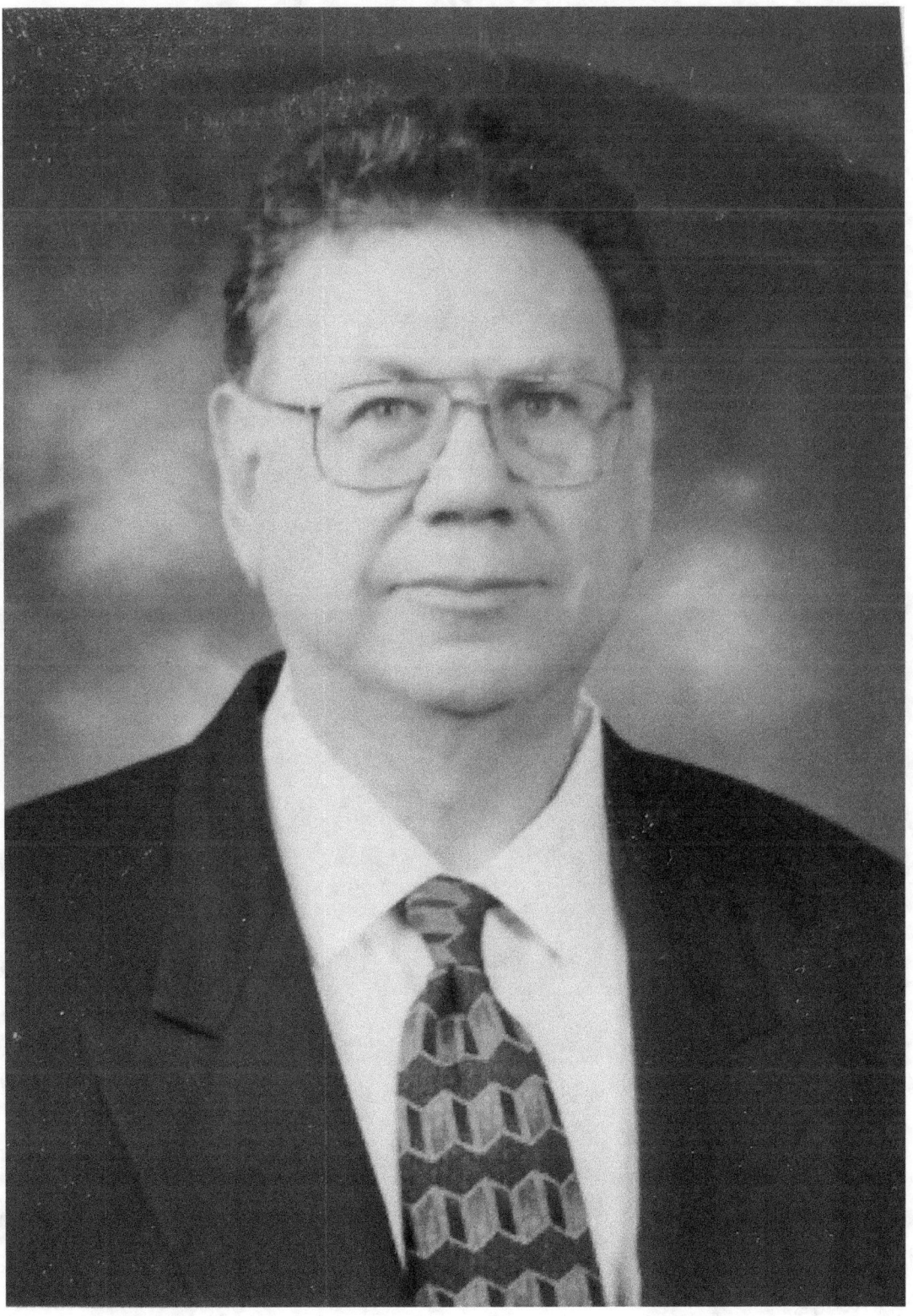

www.ingramcontent.com/pod-product-compliance
Lightning Source LLC
Chambersburg PA
CBHW080913220526
45467CB00024BA/2215